NEUROSCIENCE RESEARCH PROGRESS

PARAPLEGIA

CLINICAL CHARACTERISTICS, PREVALENCE AND TREATMENT OUTCOMES

NEUROSCIENCE RESEARCH PROGRESS

Additional books in this series can be found on Nova's website under the Series tab.

Additional e-books in this series can be found on Nova's website under the e-book tab.

NEUROSCIENCE RESEARCH PROGRESS

PARAPLEGIA

CLINICAL CHARACTERISTICS, PREVALENCE AND TREATMENT OUTCOMES

AGNES A. HOLLOWAY
EDITOR

New York

Library of Congress Cataloging-in-Publication Data

ISBN: 978-1-63482-465-1
Library of Congress Control Number: 2015934864

Published by Nova Science Publishers, Inc. † New York

Contents

PREFACE

In the last 20 years, fundamental research to repair the spinal cord has yielded positive results and today, there is real hope that a cure might be found for the treatment of spinal injuries. This has only been possible because in the last 70 years, patients with a traumatic injury of the spinal cord have been kept alive through conservative forms of treatment and returned to useful independent lives. It is salutary at this stage to look at how this conservative treatment developed. This book begins by providing a history of the treatment of spinal cord injuries and continues by examining the pertinent epidemiology, injury characteristics, and outcomes of spinal cord injury in children. It also discusses anaesthetic management of patients with chronic spinal cord injury; morphological changes of toenails in hemiplegia; and spasticity.

Chapter 1 - Injuries of the spine giving rise to paraplegia have been known since antiquity. There were excellent descriptions of the condition but the patients inevitably died within a few days of injury from pressure sores and urinary sepsis. The first effective spinal unit was established by Wilhelm Wagner (1848-1900) in Germany at the end of the 19th century at a small accident hospital at Königshutte. Wagner founded the spinal unit to treat the many injured miners who had sustained spinal injuries as a result of the collapse of tunnels. Patients were turned regularly and their bladders were drained so that early death from pressure sores and urinary tract infections could be avoided. The unit was so successful that some patients were discharged home but when Wagner died, the unit closed down.

The First World War, with an unprecedented number of casualties, showed that the existing methods of treatment were unsatisfactory, there was no triage and wounded soldiers were admitted indiscriminately to general military hospitals. Consequently, specialised units were established by all the belligerents for the treatment of abdominal wounds, for orthopaedic and plastic surgery and for spinal injuries.

Soldiers of the Central Powers suffering a spinal injury were treated in Vienna, Tübingen, Leipzig, Berlin and Breslau by a number.

France and Britain set up spinal units but the meticulous treatment pioneered in Germany whereby nursing staff and physiotherapists worked as a team with the doctors was not followed and the mortality was much higher. Marburg in Austria recorded 50 deaths out of a 150 (33% mortality) compared to a mortality of 82% in France and 65% in the UK. When the war ended, the flow of injured soldiers ceased and the military hospitals and spinal units closed down. The treatment of chronic spinal injury patients in France and the United Kingdom was unsatisfactory despite French attempts at rehabilitation. In Britain, paralysed patients were treated by orthopaedic surgeons in general and voluntary hospitals, there were very few doctors trained in rehabilitation.

The situation in the United States during the First World War was rather different. The USA did not enter the war until 1917 and owing to the great distances involved, their casualties with a spinal injury did not survive transport to the USA and spinal units were not founded. In 1936, Donald Munro (1889-1973) opened a specialised spinal unit at the Massachusetts General Hospital. Stimulated by the teaching of Frazier, Munro set up an experimental unit for the treatment of spinal cord injuries, funded by the Rockefeller Foundation. He was the first to demonstrate that spinal cord injury was not fatal but could be treated. He published extensively from 1936 onwards. His paper written in 1943 laid the foundation for the modern treatment of spinal injuries. His views are dogmatic and forceful. He maintained that by meticulous care of the patient and prevention of pressure sores, if the patient had a good pair of arms, he or she could be returned to a useful, independent existence.

In the United Kingdom, at the outset of the Second World War, spinal units were set up but they were unsatisfactory as there were no facilities, no doctors devoted exclusively to the care of the patients until Ludwig Guttmann was appointed as the only full-time Resident Medical Officer to Stoke Mandeville Hospital in 1944 that the situation changed. He instituted a Prussian regime in the Foerster tradition of medicine. He trained and supervised the auxiliary and nursing staff and carried out the catheterisation himself; he did not accept the English hierarchical system of visiting consultants giving orders and departing. He was ever present and took overall responsibility for all aspects of the patient's care. He showed by example that these patients could be successfully treated and his methods and ideas received acknowledgement and were adopted throughout Europe and the former British Empire.

In the USA, owing to a lack of a health service, Munro's doctrine could only be applied in the Veteran Hospitals. The rest of the population did not receive specialised care. In Germany, the Nazis were opposed to the rehabilitation of people with a disability and although the work had been initiated there by Wagner, the treatment of spinal injury did not evolve.

In France, owing to the occupation by the Nazis, their fine neurological tradition could not be continued and it is only well after the Second World War that Guttmann's doctrine prevailed throughout Europe and spinal units were established.

Chapter 2 - Spinal cord injury in the pediatric population is a relatively uncommon but devastating injury. Such injuries in this age group demonstrate numerous significant differences from such injuries in adults. Such differences include patterns and causes of injury, treatment algorithms, and rehabilitation potential. These carry significant implications for evaluation, treatment, and rehabilitation of these patients. In this chapter the authors review the causes and patterns of injury as well as an overview of treatment and outcomes in this population.

Chapter 3 - Increasing numbers of patients with spinal cord injury (SCI) present for surgery or intrapartum care. A higher survival of these patients has lead to an increased prevalence and an increment in patients presenting for elective surgery. Managing these patients supposes a challenge to the anaesthesiologist.

Selection of a proper anaesthesia technique must prevent essentially autonomic hyperreflexia (AH), which may occur mainly with complete lesions above T7 (incidence of 85% in those patients), as it is more frequent in patients with higher lesions. Likelihood of triggering AH is essential to choose an anaesthetic technique. This condition consists on massive autonomic response caused by stimuli below the level of the injury, mainly pelvic visceral stimulation. Up to 82% of AH episodes are caused by bladder distension. Cutaneous and proprioceptive stimuli are less commonly responsible for this phenomenon. Surgery is a potent stimulus that could also provoque this condition, mostly in patients with previous history of AH or cervical lesions. Urological surgery is the most frequent procedure causing it.

Patients with frequent spasms normally require anaesthesia to undergo surgery as they are frequently triggered by proprioceptive and cutaneous stimuli, including surgical stimulus.

Many patients with low and complete lesions could undergo surgery without anaesthesia under the level of the lesion if AH is unlikely to occur and they are no troubled by daily spasms.

If anaesthesia is indicated, both general and regional anaesthesia could be used. Due to a reduction in lean tissue mass because of muscular atrophy the volume of distribution for intravenous agents is diminished. Succinilcholine, as depolirising neuromuscular blocking agent, should not be used in the early phase of SCI with the exception of the first 72h.

Regional anaesthesia, mainly spinal anaesthesia, prevents AH and spasms but it may be difficult to assess the level of the block and to perform the technique due to previous spinal surgery or bone deformities. Spinal anaesthesia normally provides haemodynamic stability. Epidural anaesthesia may also be achieved, but it is less predictable as the epidural space is normally distorted in these patients.

AH is also a severe complication during pregnancy, labour and delivery. Epidural anaesthesia impedes the occurrence of AH with variable success. If the risk of AH is high, an epidural catheter may be placed before labour, and maintained up to 5 days after delivery, when the risk of developing AH has diminished.

Chapter 4 - Nails have numerous functions. Fingernails are important for protecting the distal phalanges, enhancing tactile discrimination, and performing fine manipulation. They are also used for scratching and grooming. Toenails protect the distal toes and contribute to pedal biomechanics. Thus, nails are frequently exposed on a daily basis to physical stimuli such as counter pressure and shear force. The author's recent studies revealed that mechanical forces may have a particularly pronounced effect on nail configuration, and thus may be involved in the development of nail deformities. One such deformity is pincer nail, which is defined as the transverse overcurvature of the nail plate that increases along the longitudinal axis. The known causative factors of pincer nail include heredity, inappropriate nail cutting, and, most commonly, poorly fitting shoes that impose inappropriate physical forces on the nail. However, the author's extensive clinical experience shows that patients with hemiplegia also frequently develop pincer nail on the palsied side, which receives weaker mechanical forces on a daily basis than the non-palsied side. At present, however, this phenomenon is poorly documented and understood.

This chapter reviews the effect of mechanical force on nail configuration and introduces the author's studies on the morphological changes of the toenails in patients with hemiplegia.

When the curvature of the great toenails on the palsied and non-palsied sides of subjects with hemiplegia was measured, the great toenail on the palsied side was found to be significantly more curved than the great toenail on the non-palsied side. This phenomenon was also observed in the mouse model of hemiplegia, which was generated by cutting the sciatic nerve in the left hin dleg of each mouse to create a denervated leg. One month after the operation, the denervated and innervated hind legs were evaluated macroscopically and histologically. The third toenails of the denervated legs were significantly more curved in the short and long axis than the third toenails of the innervated legs.

Understanding the relationship between mechanical force and nail configuration could revolutionize the treatment of nail deformities. This relationship suggests that nail deformities could be prevented and treated by eliminating excessive mechanical forces, by increasing mechanical forces, or by limiting the inherent tendency of the nail to curve, which counteracts daily downward mechanical forces. An example of the latter approach is softening the nail by applying an external preparation or thinning the nail with a nail rasp. The authors hope that the information contained in this review will help to inform and initiate future experimentation on the roles that mechanical forces play in the functions of our bodies, including our nails.

Chapter 5 - Spasticity is characterized by a velocity-dependent increase in tonic stretch reflexes with exaggerated tendon jerks, resulting from hyperexcitability of the stretch reflex. It is a common complication affecting about 67% of the patients with spinal cord injury. Problematic spasticity occurs in 40-60% of these patients. When the injury is acute, muscle tone is flaccid with hyporeflexia (spinal shock) before the appearance of spasticity.

Muscle tone is maintained by regulation of stretch reflex arc which is balanced between the inhibitory influences by corticospinal tract and dorsal reticulospinal tract, and the facilitatory influences (on extensor tone) by medial reticulospinal and verstibulospinal tract (supraspinal control). Mechanism of spasticity is commonly explained by the combination of the following neurophysiological phenomena.

1) Presynaptic inhibition of Ia afferent terminals.
2) Disynaptic reciproval Ia inhibition from muscle spindle Ia afferents from the antagonist muscles.
3) Recurrent inhibition via Renshaw cells.
4) Non-reciprocal Ib inhibition from Golgi tendon organs.
5) Inhibition from muscle spindle group II afferents

Clinically, spasticity may be of different types due to involvement of different descending pathways. Depending on the predominant involvement of phasic (dynamic) or tonic (static) components of muscle stretch reflexes, the spasticity may be phasic or tonic. It can be separated into sub-definitions.

(1) Intrinsic tonic spasticity (manifesting as increased tone),
(2) Intrinsic phasic spasticity (manifesting as tendon hyper-reflexia and clonus) and
(3) Extrinsic spasticity manifesting as spasms

Spasticity is a clinical diagnosis. Measurement methods can be divided into clinical methods, biomechanical methods and electrophysiological methods. Spasticity is disabling and, if left untreated or sub-optimally treated, may lead to consequences, such as muscle shortening, contracture, limb deformity, altered body mechanics, loading on pressure points.

The successful management of spasticity can be a therapeutic challenge. Spasticity can assist weakened legs, permit transfer ability, and improve bed mobility. Therefore all spastic patients do not need treatments. It should be treated when it causes pain,difficulty in performing daily living activities, impaired mobility, poor joint positioning, increased risk of contracture and skin breakdown.

The patient, caregiver, and healthcare professionals should agree about the treatment goals. The patient's age, preferences, and ability to comply with treatment need to be considered on the choice of treatment. The treatment of spasticity is usually initiated with the most conservative treatments that have the fewest risks. Treatment options include non-pharmacological, pharmacological and surgical interventions.

In: Paraplegia
Editor: Agnes A. Holloway
ISBN: 978-1-63482-465-1

Chapter 1

THE HISTORY OF THE TREATMENT OF SPINAL CORD INJURIES

John Russell Silver, MD
Emeritus Consultant, Stoke Mandeville Hospital, UK

ABSTRACT

Injuries of the spine giving rise to paraplegia have been known since antiquity. There were excellent descriptions of the condition but the patients inevitably died within a few days of injury from pressure sores and urinary sepsis (see figure 1). The first effective spinal unit was established by Wilhelm Wagner (1848-1900) in Germany at the end of the 19th century at a small accident hospital at Königshutte. Wagner founded the spinal unit to treat the many injured miners who had sustained spinal injuries as a result of the collapse of tunnels. Patients were turned regularly and their bladders were drained so that early death from pressure sores and urinary tract infections could be avoided. The unit was so successful that some patients were discharged home but when Wagner died, the unit closed down.

The First World War, with an unprecedented number of casualties, showed that the existing methods of treatment were unsatisfactory, there was no triage and wounded soldiers were admitted indiscriminately to general military hospitals. Consequently, specialised units were established by all the belligerents for the treatment of abdominal wounds, for orthopaedic and plastic surgery and for spinal injuries.

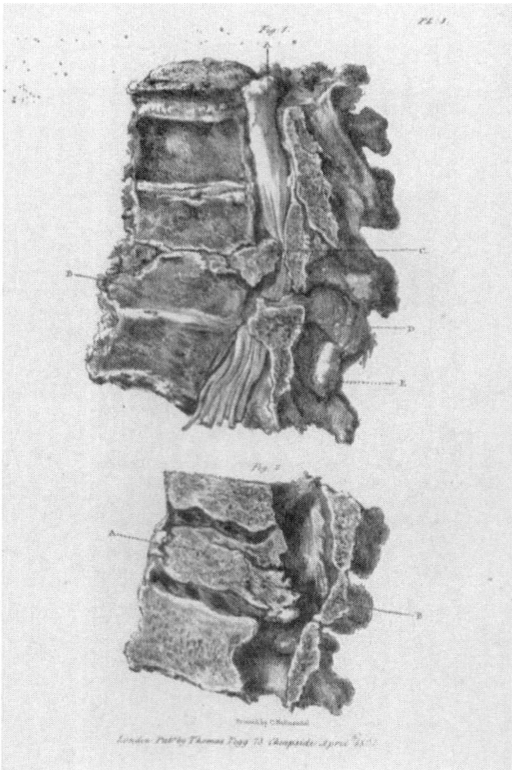

Figure 1. This beautifully drawn picture of the vertebral column by Sir Charles Bell shows the pathology of spinal cord injury. (Bell, 1924) The pathology of such injury was appreciated long before any treatment emerged. Reproduced by kind permission of the Wellcome Library London.

Soldiers of the Central Powers suffering a spinal injury were treated in Vienna, Tübingen, Leipzig, Berlin and Breslau by a number.

France and Britain set up spinal units but the meticulous treatment pioneered in Germany whereby nursing staff and physiotherapists worked as a team with the doctors was not followed and the mortality was much higher. Marburg in Austria recorded 50 deaths out of a 150 (33% mortality) compared to a mortality of 82% in France and 65% in the UK. When the war ended, the flow of injured soldiers ceased and the military hospitals and spinal units closed down. The treatment of chronic spinal injury patients in France and the United Kingdom was unsatisfactory despite French attempts at rehabilitation. In Britain, paralysed patients were treated by orthopaedic surgeons in general and voluntary hospitals, there were very few doctors trained in rehabilitation.

The situation in the United States during the First World War was rather different. The USA did not enter the war until 1917 and owing to the great distances involved, their casualties with a spinal injury did not survive transport to the USA and spinal units were not founded. In 1936, Donald Munro (1889-1973) opened a specialised spinal unit at the Massachusetts General Hospital. Stimulated by the teaching of Frazier, Munro set up an experimental unit for the treatment of spinal cord injuries, funded by the Rockefeller Foundation. He was the first to demonstrate that spinal cord injury was not fatal but could be treated. He published extensively from 1936 onwards. His paper written in 1943 laid the foundation for the modern treatment of spinal injuries. His views are dogmatic and forceful. He maintained that by meticulous care of the patient and prevention of pressure sores, if the patient had a good pair of arms, he or she could be returned to a useful, independent existence.

In the United Kingdom, at the outset of the Second World War, spinal units were set up but they were unsatisfactory as there were no facilities, no doctors devoted exclusively to the care of the patients until Ludwig Guttmann was appointed as the only full-time Resident Medical Officer to Stoke Mandeville Hospital in 1944 that the situation changed. He instituted a Prussian regime in the Foerster tradition of medicine. He trained and supervised the auxiliary and nursing staff and carried out the catheterisation himself; he did not accept the English hierarchical system of visiting consultants giving orders and departing. He was ever present and took overall responsibility for all aspects of the patient's care. He showed by example that these patients could be successfully treated and his methods and ideas received acknowledgement and were adopted throughout Europe and the former British Empire.

In the USA, owing to a lack of a health service, Munro's doctrine could only be applied in the Veteran Hospitals. The rest of the population did not receive specialised care. In Germany, the Nazis were opposed to the rehabilitation of people with a disability and although the work had been initiated there by Wagner, the treatment of spinal injury did not evolve.

In France, owing to the occupation by the Nazis, their fine neurological tradition could not be continued and it is only well after the Second World War that Guttmann's doctrine prevailed throughout Europe and spinal units were established.

INTRODUCTION

In the last 20 years, fundamental research to repair the spinal cord has yielded positive results and today, there is real hope that a cure might be found for the treatment of spinal injuries. This has only been possible because in the last 70 years, patients with a traumatic injury of the spinal cord have been kept alive through conservative forms of treatment and returned to useful independent lives. It is salutary at this stage to look at how this conservative treatment developed. This chapter focuses on the pioneering role of German medicine in the treatment of spinal injuries.

The development of spinal injury units during the Second World War was one of the success stories of neurological rehabilitation, demonstrating that patients could be kept alive and returned to a useful life. The successful treatment of spinal injuries is attributed to Donald Munro (1936, USA) and Ludwig Guttmann (1944, UK); yet Dr. Kluger, a retired German surgeon, has suggested that the treatment of spinal injuries originated not in the United States or Britain but in Germany before the First World War. He argued that this knowledge was suppressed and forgotten. This chapter explores this argument further and with particular focus on Ludwig Guttmann's contribution. I worked with Ludwig Guttmann for many years, initially as his registrar in 1956 and subsequently from 1962-5 as a senior research registrar and kept in contact with him until his death. Consequently, I have a unique insight into his background, research and clinical methods.

Historical Background

The first effective spinal unit was established by Wilhelm Wagner (1848–1900) at the end of the 19th century in Königshütte in Germany. Wagner founded the unit to treat injured miners who had sustained spinal injuries as a result of collapsed tunnels. Patients were turned regularly and their bladder drained so that early deaths from pressure sores and urinary tract infection could be avoided. Some patients were discharged home but after Wagner's death the unit closed down. Emil Theodor Kocher (1841–1917), using the same principles, treated spinal injury patients in Bern, Switzerland. Wagner and Kocher's textbooks became the standard references for the treatment of spinal injuries during the First World War. Just as the congregation of injured coal miners led Wagner to found a spinal unit, so the First World War showed that the existing methods of treatment were unsatisfactory as there was no triage and vast numbers of casualties were admitted indiscriminately to general military hospitals. Consequently, all the belligerents established specialised units for the treatment of abdominal wounds, for orthopaedic and plastic surgery, and for spinal injuries.

THE TREATMENT OF SPINAL INJURIES DURING THE FIRST WORLD WAR BY THE CENTRAL POWERS, AND THE UNITED KINGDOM

Germany

Patients were treated in Vienna by O. Marburg (1874–1948), E. Ranzi (1875–1939) and A. Eiselberg (1860–1939), in Tübingen Leipzig by C. Perthes (1869–1927) and Paul Fragenheim (1876–1930), in Berlin by F. Krause (1856–1937), A. Borchard (1864–1940) and R. Cassirer (1868–1925) and in Breslau by Otfrid Foerster (1873–1941) and Sigmund Weil (1881–1961).

Methods of Treatment

Doctors recognised that patients with spinal injuries would need lifelong care. Marburg, already a professor of neurology, established a spinal unit in Vienna with a team of specialists in urology, neurology, neurosurgery and orthopaedic surgery. He described the importance of supervising the nursing staff and monitoring the patient's bladder. He incorporated physiotherapy in his treatment regime and endeavoured to return the patients home. With Ranzi, he assessed the benefits of early surgery upon the damaged spinal cord.

The United Kingdom (UK)

At the outset of the War, the Regular Army Medical Officers ceased clinical work in order to perform an administrative role. A few doctors were recruited and consultants from the Voluntary Hospitals continued to practise in London while visiting Military Hospitals on a rotating basis. Patients were congregated at the receiving hospitals and transferred to the United Kingdom for treatment but it soon became apparent, just as in the other countries involved in the conflict, that segregation and specialisation were essential to treat head injuries, neurotrauma, spinal injuries, abdominal wounds and orthopaedic injuries.

Methods of Treatment

The lack of a coordinated approach to the treatment of spinal injuries resulted in a high mortality rate because of both the ascending infection of the renal tract and the presence of pressure sores. If they survived the battle field, soldiers with spinal injuries came under the care of Gordon Holmes (1876–1965) in the Military Field Hospitals in France and were transferred to the London Hospital under Henry Head (1861–1940) or to the King George V Hospital under Charles Charters Symonds (1852–1932). Injured officers were transferred to The Empire Hospital in London, a neurotrauma unit staffed solely by neurologists (among them George Riddoch (1888–1947), Henry Head and Samuel Kinnier Wilson (1878–1937)). The unit lacked a urologist but nevertheless, the results were better than in other hospitals. The fundamentals of treatment were recognised although these were not documented until 1924 with the publication of a Medical Research Council (MRC) instruction manual setting out the key principles of treatment.

Long-Term Medical and Social Care of Surviving Paraplegics after the War

In Germany, spinal units closed and spinal injury patients were looked after by neurologists and psychiatrists, but the standard of medicine was exceptional. Marburg returned to his professorial unit in Vienna where he treated all forms of neurological disease including paraplegia and he maintained his interest in the subject by writing the section on spinal injuries in the Handbook of Neurology. He also discussed the importance of preventing sporting injuries of the spine. In 1925, an innovative accident hospital opened in Vienna under a gifted visionary surgeon, Lorenz Böhler (1885–1973); his ideas influenced the world, in particular, the accident and emergency movement in Britain. Böhler's clinic was organised meticulously and he supervised all aspects of treatment. There was an interchange of roles whereby nurses and orderlies carried out the work that doctors would usually have undertaken, thereby providing continuity of care. This thus became the forerunner of spinal injury management. Böhler carried out all forms of rehabilitation including that of spinal injury patients. Specialisation was encouraged throughout Germany where neurology was well established as a speciality. Foerster set up a comprehensive neurological rehabilitation unit for patients with peripheral nerve injuries.

In the United Kingdom, all but one of the military hospitals closed down and doctors returned to their pre-war clinical practices in neurology. The Empire Hospital became a hotel and the King George V Hospital became a warehouse. An exception was the Military Orthopaedic Hospital in Oxford, which was bought by Lord Morris and became the Nuffield Orthopaedic Hospital. Long-term survivors were admitted to the Royal Star and Garter Home where doctors tried to rehabilitate them with physiotherapy but most patients languished there with renal sepsis and pressure sores. The urologist J. Thomson Walker (1871–1937) visited the Royal Star and Garter Home infrequently and Riddoch and Head never went there at all. Civilians were cared for in General Hospitals where the facilities were lacking and treatment was desultory. The Royal Colleges and the consultants at the Voluntary Hospitals opposed specialisation. Paralysed patients were treated in the first instance by the neurologists at The National Hospital for Nervous Diseases at Queen Square whose interest lay in diagnosis not treatment and there were no beds for long-term rehabilitation. Neurologists were few and far between; they had a low status in the hospital hierarchy and were rarely on the staff of the Voluntary Hospitals. The long-term treatment of paralysed patients was delegated to orthopaedic surgeons who also suffered from a low status within the profession. Most did not hold an appointment at a Voluntary or General Hospital; they worked in specialist hospitals including The Agnes Hunt and Robert Jones Hospital at Oswestry, nursing homes and spas.

The Pre-Eminence of German Medicine and Its Influence on the Treatment of Spinal Injuries

Rehabilitation and the development of spinal injury treatment did not arise as an isolated phenomenon in Germany; it was a reflection of the high status of medicine in society. There was an integrated approach to medicine with professorial departments based on research and teaching. Doctors came from all over the world for training.

Rehabilitation

Germany was a pioneer in the field of neurology and psychiatry and was the birthplace of neuropathology. Doctors had laid the foundation for rehabilitation treatment and Germany continued its long-standing tradition of exercise therapy in between the wars in several innovative rehabilitation departments in Germany and Austria. Heinrich Frenkel (1860–1931), a spa doctor in Switzerland, pioneered rehabilitation by teaching his tabetic patients to walk, using their eyes to compensate for the loss of position sense. Trained by Frenkel and Carl Wernicke (1848–1905), Foerster's professional thesis was on coordination and he set up the first department of neurology separate from that of psychiatry in Breslau. As Wernicke's assistant, he tried to establish a scientific basis for physical rehabilitation and physiotherapy: 'he caused the lame to walk and the blind to see'. His particular interest in peripheral nerve injuries started during the First World War when he treated 4,748 such patients and operated on 775. When he returned to his neurosurgical department in Breslau after the War, he treated all forms of neurological disease including spinal injuries. Like Böhler, he recognised the importance of continuity of care and he saw each patient as an experimental model. He examined them before starting treatment and he monitored the results. He investigated the recovery of peripheral nerve function through studies on sweating and thermoregulation. Crucially, Foerster trained Ludwig Guttmann in the management of peripheral nerve injuries and it was this rigorous Prussian training that influenced Ludwig Guttmann (see figure 2).

During his time working under Foerster, Guttmann made a significant finding. He realised that the clinical testing of sensation using pin prick, touch, hot and cold and electrical stimulation was too subjective. He observed the correlation between the recovery of sensation and the recovery of sweating. This had been measured previously using the starch iodine method, where starch turned blue when moistened by sweat. Guttmann developed a new and more sensitive method using quinizarin, a dye that also changed colour to purple when wet and he published his results in Germany.

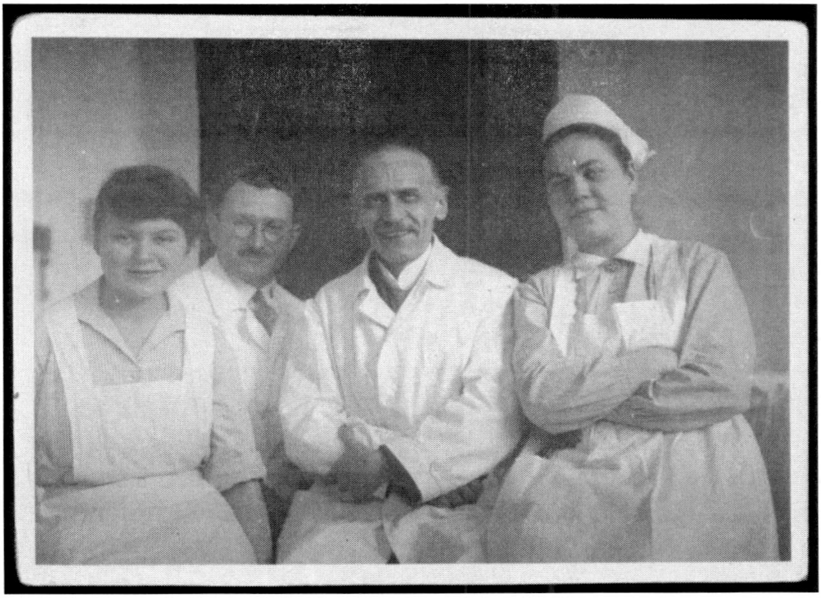

Figure 2. Otfrid Foerster with Ludwig Guttmann and nurses in Breslau. Reproduced by kind permission of the Wellcome Library London.

LEAVING GERMANY

Within weeks of Hitler coming to power in 1933, the new Nazi racial laws resulted in the dismissal of all Jews from official positions. Jewish doctors were dismissed from state hospitals and allowed to treat only Jewish patients; they were no longer called physicians but '*Krankenbehandler*', a derogatory and demeaning term which effectively stripped them of professional status. Guttmann was expelled from his job as Foerster's first assistant and his professorship was withdrawn. He took the post of neurologist and neurosurgeon at the Jewish Hospital in Breslau where he was able to continue his research work. He described how 'we have become outlaws, outcasts of the community'. For Jews, life in Germany had degenerated into a nightmare. The 1938 '*Kristallnacht*' heralded a violent pogrom against the Jewish community in Germany and many injured Jews were admitted to the Jewish Hospital in Breslau. Later that year, Guttmann, by now an internationally recognised neurosurgeon, was invited to Lisbon to treat a patient, but his family's passports had been confiscated by the Nazis. Portugal's dictator, Dr. Salazar, personally intervened with the Nazi regime and Guttmann's passport was returned to him by Joachim von Ribbentrop, Germany's Foreign Minister. On his return journey, Guttmann went to London and met a representative of the Academic Assistance Council (AAC), known today as the Council for Assisting Refugee Academics (CARA), to discuss the possibility of leaving Germany for England. Guttmann had already written to Professor Hugh Cairns (1896–1952) (neurosurgeon and Professor of Surgery at Oxford University) and had been offered a voluntary (unpaid) research assistant position. The AAC agreed to support Guttmann with an initial grant of £250 per annum for six months on condition that Guttmann's aunt, Mme B Tournel, who lived in France, would support the family thereafter. A year later, Guttmann and his family were granted a visa to go to England for three days. Guttmann realised that his only hope was to emigrate with his family. With the AAC's assistance Guttmann left Germany on 14 March 1939 with his wife Else and their two children aged eight and four, with only a few German marks in their possession. A day after the Guttmann family reached Dover, Hitler marched into Prague and occupied Czechoslovakia.

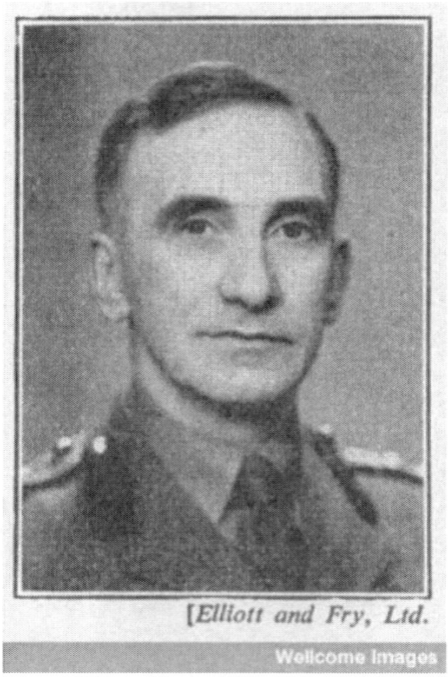

Figure 3. Brigadier George Riddoch. Reproduced by kind permission of the Wellcome Library London.

Provision of Spinal Units in the UK

The lessons learned in the First World War about medical treatment were applied during the Second World War and medical provision was planned in anticipation of a large number of casualties. At the outset of the war George Riddoch (1888–1947), who had treated patients with spinal injuries at the Empire Hospital in London during the previous war, was appointed Chairman of the Peripheral Nerve Injuries Committee of the Medical Research Council (later called the Nerve Injuries Committee) (see figure 3). It also had responsibility for spinal injuries. This committee advised the Emergency Medical Service. Many servicemen with peripheral nerve injuries also had orthopaedic injuries and, for this reason, they were treated at three designated orthopaedic hospitals in England: The Nuffield Hospital in Oxford, Otley Park Emergency Hospital in Chertsey, Surrey, and Winwick Emergency Hospital in Warrington, Lancashire. Scotland was served by two units: Gogarburn, near Edinburgh, and Killearn, near Glasgow.

Guttmann's Research at Oxford

When Guttmann arrived in Oxford, he began non-clinical work in the Nuffield Department of Neurosurgery at the Radcliffe Infirmary, under Hugh Cairns. He could not practise neurosurgery because he did not have a registerable medical qualification. Foreign doctors were expected to take an examination in anatomy and physiology and undertake two years of clinical work before sitting examinations. Guttmann's neurosurgical training under Foerster was not acceptable to Cairns because he had not trained under Harvey Cushing (1869-1939). Cushing founded modern neurosurgery. His techniques and training were the recognised standard and virtually all neurosurgeons were trained by him directly and then in turn imparted this knowledge to their pupils so that all neurosurgery practised in the world today is in 'Cushing's tradition of neurosurgery'. Guttmann was encouraged instead to take part in on-going research on peripheral nerve injuries. He had already received a thorough training in experimental physiology from Foerster and developed his quinizarin sweating technique which was essential to study the progress of nerve regeneration.

St Hugh's College, Oxford

The treatment of head injuries was limited and required specialist treatment facilities. In 1940, Cairns, Riddoch (neurologist to the Army) and Sir Charles Symonds (1890–1978) (neurologist for the Royal Air Force) set up a neurological hospital for head injuries at St Hugh's College, Oxford; a women's college put at their disposal during the war. St Hugh's became a superb combined neurological/neurosurgical unit with 450 beds at its peak. It was staffed jointly by Army and Air Force personnel: Cairns (Army) was the neurosurgeon, Derek Denny-Brown (1901–1981) (Air Force) and William Ritchie Russell (1903–1980) were the neurologists and Dorothy Stuart Russell (1895–1983), the pathologist. Denny-Brown later became Professor of Neurology at Harvard in Boston. Denis Williams (1908–1990) and many other neurologists and neurosurgeons worked there. A total of 13,000 servicemen and women were treated there and it became the training centre for the mobile neurosurgical teams where surgeons and nurses were trained to treat head injuries close to the front line. Contemporary papers document the research that was carried out on the management, treatment and transport of patients with head injuries, the long-term studies done on epilepsy and the use of electroencephalograms (EEG).

The Nerve Injury Centre, Wingfield Morris Orthopaedic Hospital

In 1940, because of his experience in working with Foerster treating victims of the First World War, Guttmann was invited by Mr (later Sir) Herbert Seddon (1903–1977), the director of the newly founded peripheral nerve injury centre at the Wingfield Morris Orthopaedic Hospital, to join the team, which included Ruth Bowden and Donal Brooks. The unit integrated all aspects of treatment: the diagnosis, surgical repair, subsequent rehabilitation by physiotherapists, followed by a full rehabilitation programme to enable the patients to return to work. The outcome of treatment was carefully documented with Riddoch's protocols. Seddon repeated Head and Rivers' work on cutting the lateral cutaneous nerve of the arm. He had his own lateral cutaneous nerve of the thigh crushed and Guttmann tested it for recovery of sensation. Guttmann was particularly interested in the unit's organisation and how patients' progress was documented. He brought his own clinical experience and carried out experiments on sweating at St Hugh's Hospital.

Experimentation

The main issues encountered by the physicians treating wartime injuries were the regeneration of peripheral nerves after injury, whether unmyelinated fibres grew faster than myelinated fibres, and neuroma formation and its inhibition. The team investigated the biochemical conditions which control nerve fibre growth and made useful surgical improvements to aid nerve regeneration. They sought to accelerate the repair of peripheral nerves severed by injury. In collaboration with Peter Medawar (1915–1987), JZ Young (1907–1997) developed a 'glue' from plasma to rejoin small peripheral nerves. This method was eventually modified and used during surgery. Guttmann used his experience in plotting sensory loss to follow the re-innervation of skin in rabbits in order to establish whether the first fibres grew in from adjacent areas or were regenerated from the main trunk. He worked with Young and Medawar on the rate of regeneration of nerve fibres and the chemical inhibition of regeneration and neuroma formation. With Ernst Gutmann (1910–1978), a refugee from Czechoslovakia (and no relation to Ludwig Guttmann), and Graham Weddell (1908–1990), he demonstrated the growth of fibres from surrounding areas. Guttmann's work with Ernst Gutmann on the effect of denervation on muscle atrophy showed that, with stimulation of the nerve, the bulk of the muscle was preserved so that if recovery subsequently occurred, the muscle could be re-innervated and not suffer from fibrosis. Guttmann went on to use this technique with paraplegic patients. They also demonstrated that galvanic stimulation of the muscles, if started immediately after injury, reduced the rate of atrophy; he applied this technique to paraplegic patients when he came to Stoke Mandeville. Guttmann's expertise led Riddoch to invite him to lecture to the neurology section of the Royal Society of Medicine in 1941, where he set out his principles of rehabilitation, his experience with Foerster, and the methods he would later use to treat paraplegic patients. Guttmann was very unhappy in Oxford and thirsted for hand-on clinical experience and he would achieve this with the intervention of George Riddoch who was so impressed with Guttmann's work that in 1944 he invited him to set up the spinal unit at Stoke Mandeville telling him 'you will have to start from scratch'. Only when Riddoch appointed Guttmann to take charge at Stoke Mandeville did an effective unit emerge in the United

Kingdom. Riddoch supported his work and encouraged him to submit his research on autonomic dysreflexia. He personally sponsored Guttmann and organised a grant from the Medical Research Council to support his work on autonomic dysreflexia. He helped him obtain equipment for his research and regularly visited the unit. Riddoch, as the foremost neurologist in the country, personally saw that Guttmann, a foreigner, a Jew and an outsider, should be accepted by the establishment. Guttmann later acknowledged this support by dedicating his book on the comprehensive treatment of spinal injuries to Riddoch.

Guttmann's Research at Stoke Mandeville and the Oxford Physiology Department

Guttmann treated patients at Stoke Mandeville, but still wanted to carry out research. He requested three half days a week to continue his studies on the physiology and pathology of sweating, using his quinizarin method. In his 1944 research application, he described how the segregation of spinal cord and spinal root injuries in a single centre would allow a systematic study of the correlation of the disturbance of sweating and sensibility during the various stages after injury as well as other functions such as heat regulation, mass reflexes and oculo-pupillary function. He described how his quinizarin method was used as an indicator of sweat gland activity and he designed a special chamber for the thermo-regulatory sweat test. Guttmann recognised that sweating was only one manifestation of autonomic function and he began to study blood flow and its control with Roger Gilliatt (1922-1991), then a medical student and later one of the most influential neurologists of his generation. Guttmann identified the correlation between sweating and blood flow but, at that time, blood pressure was not recorded, and so he was not yet aware of the significance of the overall cardiovascular changes. However, as early as April 1944, Guttmann noticed that in three patients with lesions at T3, 4 and 5, when their bladders were washed out their faces and necks became flushed, their noses seemed to be blocked, their heart rates decreased and they complained of severe headaches. In order to study temperature changes produced by bladder distension in spite of complete cord lesions, Guttmann asked David Whitteridge (1912–1994), with whom he had been working in Oxford, to bring a multiple skin thermometer. Subsequently, a portable plethysmograph was used for recording blood flow and the volume of pulsation of the toe. In the first patient, the skin temperature went up as expected in the head and neck but went down in the legs and it was obvious that a major redistribution of blood flow had taken place. In the second patient, they measured blood pressure which rose from 90/60 mmHg to 220/140 mmHg. Guttmann and Whitteridge set up a collaborative study to assess patients with lesions at all levels. They showed how, although vasoconstriction occurred in the toes of all patients, blood pressure remained steady in patients with lesions at and below T7, and rose sharply in patients with lesions above T6. This was a viscero-cutaneous reflex triggered by distension of the bladder. This reaction could also be triggered by distension of the rectum, the intestine and the uterus. The stimulus spread as far as it could in the isolated cord and excited sympathetic vasoconstrictor fibres in the lateral column. With low lesions, vasoconstriction occurred first in the legs followed by vasodilatation in the upper half of the body and slowing of the pulse. With lesions above T6, vasoconstriction occurred in more widely spread parts of the body and was evident in the hands. The regulatory mechanism still produced slowing of the heart, but the vascular territory was too small for effective vasodilatation. The effects observed are perversions of the homeostatic mechanisms controlling the circulation. To study the overall cardiac output, Guttmann, Cunningham, Whitteridge and Wyndham used the conventional acetylene method, but the cardiac output did not change. These studies are seminal to our understanding of autonomic dysreflexia. Wyndham returned to South Africa where he studied heat regulation in miners. He returned briefly to Stoke Mandeville Hospital and collaborated with Guttmann and myself in studying heat regulation in tetraplegic patients.

THE NATIONAL SPINAL INJURY CENTRE AT STOKE MANDEVILLE HOSPITAL

The previous part of this paper documents where Ludwig Guttmann obtained his training before setting up the National Spinal Injuries Centre. In 1944 Guttmann was appointed Resident Medical Officer in charge of the spinal unit. He had to leave his wife and family in Oxford as the children were settled in schools. He lacked equipment and medical staff and the nurses and the orderlies (who were from the Army) had to be trained. He set about implementing the lessons he had learned from treating peripheral nerve injuries patients to the treatment of paraplegic patients. Ludwig Guttmann was a product of the German university system with its emphasis on research. At the beginning of the 20th century, German and Austrian medicine had gained an outstanding reputation in leading the world in the study of clinical diagnosis, therapy and research. Their contribution to scientific research and clinical practice was in contrast to Great Britain where the emphasis was on bedside teaching. There were few centres of clinical research apart from the lonely beacons of the Hammersmith Hospital and the Medical Research Council. Full-time research posts were few and far between and lacked status. Consequently, motivated medical and postgraduate students travelled to Germany to obtain further training and a doctorate to further their scientific career since this was not possible in the United Kingdom.

Foerster taught Guttmann how to examine and treat paralysed patients. He studied the patient before starting treatment in order to determine the nature of the problem. Similarly, Guttmann was meticulous in seeing every patient on admission, sometimes in the ambulance or on a stretcher. He directed the investigations and believed in a consultant-led programme. Consequently, the first vital 48 hours were not lost. This is in contrast to the established practice in the United Kingdom where the patient would be seen initially by a junior houseman and the consultant might not see the patient for several days. Like Foerster, Guttmann had a hands-on approach.

When he was appointed in charge of Stoke Mandeville as the only doctor, he insisted that every aspect of the treatment was his responsibility. He supervised the turning of the patient in the middle of the night and undertook the catheterisations himself. Just as Foerster had congregated patients with peripheral nerve injuries, Guttmann was insistent in gathering together all the spinal injury patients under his care. He was opposed to the opening up of other spinal units in the South of England so he could have large numbers of patients for statistical analysis and research. Guttmann acknowledged in his autobiography that his experience in peripheral nerve injuries was directly applicable to the treatment of spinal injury patients. Foerster was a disciple of Duchenne and Sherrington and he realised that the paralysis was different in tabetic patients and patients with a stroke and that the spasticity could be relieved by root section. Guttmann observed this and applied it by using an alcohol block to the spinal cord. Foerster appreciated from his work with Frenkel in Switzerland that physical means of treatment in tabes, utilising the intact parts of the body and the eyes to compensate for the paralysed parts, were fundamental in treatment and Foerster published extensively on the subject. Guttmann seized on this and physiotherapy became the cornerstone of his rehabilitation treatment (see figure 4). He was fortunate that when he was appointed the School of Massage at the Middlesex Hospital was based at Stoke Mandeville Hospital and the masseurs were recruited to carry out the physiotherapy. At first they were opposed to it but later on they became enthusiasts and this served as the foundation not only of rehabilitation of the patients but also of physiotherapy in the United Kingdom. Guttmann's psychiatric training in Hamburg and his thorough grounding in neuropathology proved invaluable in organising the rehabilitation of the patients.

Guttmann, a Jewish refugee had a thorough training in Germany through looking after paralysed patients and had learned from Munro's work but his qualifications were not recognized in the UK and he was not able to practise medicine until 1944. Guttmann was a restless driven man, determined to return the patients to a meaningful life and he welcomed the opportunity to treat patients at Stoke Mandeville Hospital. He arrived in 1944, full of optimism and energy. He had gained remarkable ideas from Otfrid Foerster (1873–1941), neurologist in Germany, about physiotherapy and about operations on the spinal cord and nerve roots in order to relieve spasticity. All these factors Guttmann incorporated into his practice.

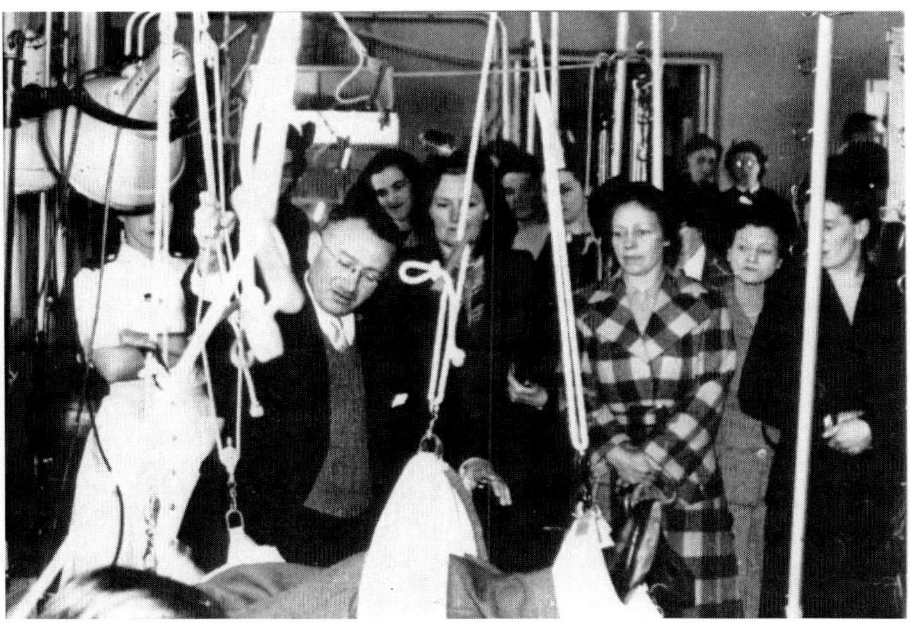

Figure 4. Ludwig Guttmann at his happiest teaching physiotherapists at Stoke Mandeville Hospital. Personal photograph Dr. John Silver reproduced with kind permission from Springer Science+Business Media B.V.

Pressure Sores

When the pressure sores were healed, he was in favour of simple surgery, opposing the skin and pulling the skin together to cover the wound to provide a healthy base. He used skin grafts for larger sores. When the skin was sound and healthy, the patients were gradually mobilized and taught how to prevent further sores by lifting themselves regularly, and how to walk with callipers.

Bladder Management

Guttmann took full responsibility for the management of the bladder, personally carrying out intermittent catheterization regularly four times a day and whenever the bladder became distended, as a surgical procedure by a doctor fully gloved and gowned with the catheter team going from patient to patient.

Physiotherapy

The immobilization following acute paraplegia led to an unfortunate series of complications, contractures of the muscles with stiff joints and deep vein thrombosis in the lower limbs. These could all be overcome by active physiotherapy (not recognized as a specialty in 1944). Guttmann was fortunate in finding that the

Middlesex School of Masseurs was based at Stoke Mandeville Hospital (the Middlesex Hospital was evacuated to Stoke Mandeville then). Initially, there was no physiotherapy department and the patients underwent physiotherapy treatment in the middle of the ward.

Rehabilitation of the Patients

Guttmann pioneered the concept in the UK of returning the patient to a useful life. Once the patients had regained the ability to look after their skin, to dress and undress themselves, transfer and be independent and manage their bladders, they were discharged from the hospital.

Research

Every patient was studied as an experiment in neuropathology. Guttmann studied the results of the paralysis of the sympathetic system because he noticed in 1944 that, when the bladder was washed out, the patient's face and neck went red and the nose seemed blocked, the heart slowed and the patient complained of severe headache. Intrigued by these changes, Guttmann worked with David Whitteridge (1912–94), Lecturer at the Physiology Department at Oxford University, studying the effects of spinal cord transaction upon the sympathetic nervous system. Guttmann went on to study postural hypotension and temperature regulation. He studied breathing by electromyography of the respiratory muscles and carried out experiments on stimulating the spinal cord with prostigmine which resulted in ejaculation and rendered the sterile patient fertile. He carried out practical research on renal function and the healing of pressure sores. He published his work, initially in a monograph of medical treatment during World War II and then in a textbook on the treatment of spinal injuries which has not been bettered to this day. He founded the International Society of Paraplegia and the Journal Paraplegia (now Spinal Cord), both of which are flourishing today.

Influence

Guttmann was an energetic man and a superb administrator who tolerated no opposition from politicians, administrators, doctors or members of staff. He insisted that every aspect of the patients' care was his responsibility (he never took a holiday). He saw patients on admission, sometimes in the ambulance or on a stretcher, weekly on the ward rounds and later in the physiotherapy and occupational therapy departments. This was in contrast to the organization in the teaching hospitals in the UK where the consultant visited once or twice a week. He imbued the whole unit with his will and dynamism. His influence was first felt on the spinal unit where patients and staff became motivated and enthusiastic but, later on, his mark was felt in other spinal units and Stoke Mandeville Hospital served as a benchmark; it was no longer acceptable for the patients in other units to have pressure sores. The Ministry of Health stated that Stoke Mandeville Hospital was the only acceptable unit. This resulted in staff being seconded to Stoke Mandeville Hospital to learn Guttmann's methods.

THE SPORTS MOVEMENT

Guttmann's other major contribution was to sports medicine. This happened soon after 1945 when Guttmann noticed patients in their wheelchairs outside the unit hitting a puck with inverted walking sticks. He jumped in a chair himself, tried it and realized that sport must be an integral part of patients' treatment.

HISTORICAL BACKGROUND

Sport improves the self-esteem of disabled people. It helps them reintegrate into society so that they can compete against other disabled persons and in some sports against able-bodied persons. Historically, the first record of disabled persons participating in sport was in the Napoleonic Wars when a team of one-armed patients at Greenwich Hospital played a team of one-legged patients at cricket. In the 19th century two one-legged amputees were each provided with a wooden leg and held a walking race during a sports festival at Newmarket Heath, to the enthusiasm of the spectators. During World War I volleyball was introduced in the UK for persons with amputations, and non-competitive swimming was being used as a method of rehabilitation. In Germany sport was developed for blind persons and for those with amputations. This started during World War I and between the World Wars techniques were well developed and competitive meetings held.

Karl Gebhardt (1897–1948) used sport for rehabilitation in Germany before World War II. The British Legion visited his clinic in 1936 in an effort to establish friendships with German veterans of World War I: 'The aim of Dr. Gebhardt's training is to make the amputated case so fit and strong and so active with his one leg and one arm that he gets to feel as active and as efficient as the man with two legs or two arms. To this end, it is generally six months before the man receives his artificial limb. This also gives time for the stump to get hardened and to assume its final form. A temporary artificial limb is supplied but the constant use of this is not encouraged'. Disabled persons had their own sports movement and their own Olympics. The British were predominant in tennis and soccer and at the International Games held in Nuremberg in 1931 they complained bitterly not only that the foreigners were receiving subsidies, which they were not, but that there had been cheating in their football game against Czechoslovakia. They were truly competitive sports. This movement became significant and assumed an international role. Guttmann reviewed the whole subject admirably. It is not known whether Ludwig Guttmann, who trained in Germany and was Consultant at the Royal Star and Garter Home, was aware of these sporting activities but when he established the spinal unit at Stoke Mandeville Hospital in 1944 he was treating young, vigorous soldiers and they began to participate in sporting activities on the wards. He was determined that these soldiers should not only survive but also function as fully contributing members of society. He introduced sport primarily to train the body but secondarily to revive the spirit of accomplishment and self-worth. Initially physiotherapists used sport as a form of rehabilitation. It was carried out on the wards, in the gymnasium, in the car park and on the lawns at Stoke Mandeville Hospital. It began with archery, snooker and table tennis, team sports were added later, wheelchair polo and basketball.

Competitive Sport

On 28 July 1948, 16 paralysed British ex-servicemen and women from the Royal Star and Garter Home and Stoke Mandeville Hospital engaged in an archery competition on the lawns of Stoke Mandeville Hospital. This transformed the face of sport from rehabilitation to competition. The number of athletes and the number of countries participating rose steadily and more sports were introduced. Patients with other disabilities were able to take part.

Equipment

Initially competitors used standard Travaux wheelchairs but these were heavy and difficult to manoeuvre and best suited to stationary activities such as archery. Other sports demanded adaptations. For activities that demanded mobility of the chair, such as basketball, lightweight wheelchairs (Everest and Jennings) were introduced from the USA along with basketball which Deaver had developed in the USA. Specialized devices for anchoring wheelchairs for fencing were first used in 1961 and specialized racing wheelchairs made their first appearance in the Paralympic Summer Games in Toronto in 1976. Nowadays sports wheelchairs are light, manoeuvrable and strong and rather like a sports shoe have been developed to a level that chairs are tailor made for the individual to maximize performance. Titanium and light alloys combined with creative design have led to aesthetically increased functionality. Specialized skis enable snow sports.

FACILITIES

In the early days at Stoke Mandeville Hospital the visiting teams slept in the wards, in the laboratories and in doctors' quarters, to the detriment of medical treatment. The number of athletes increased and the standard of competition improved, spurring the need for more and better facilities. Facilities suitable for recreation were not suitable for competition. Wheelchair basketball could not be played competitively on a gravel car park. It had to be moved indoors to a sports hall with a special floor. Certain sports such as swimming could not take place until the pool provided for hydrotherapy was built but this proved too small for competitive events. Competitors demanded more appropriate facilities and money was raised to build a sports stadium at Stoke Mandeville by public appeal on the understanding that the facilities would be made available to the general public. The Ministry of Health made the ground available at £1 per year rent. By September 1969 the building fund stood at £296,922 and the stadium was officially opened for the 1969 International Games. Over the years many facilities have been added. An Olympic Village was completed in time for the 1981 International Stoke Mandeville Games. The stadium was refurbished in 2003 at a cost of £10.2 million. The stadium now includes sleeping accommodation, badminton, an indoor bowling green, athletics track, multi-sports hall and swimming pool. It also serves as a conference centre with meeting rooms, a group training studio, café/bar and a crèche. Such facilities are expensive to build, run and maintain. The stadium at Stoke Mandeville now costs around £1,000,000 per year to run. It is also the headquarters of the British Wheelchair Sports Foundation, which also costs £1,000,000 a year to run. Sport for disabled persons evolved from rehabilitation to competition. The first teams to compete at Stoke Mandeville were from the UK. The idea spread and the Dutch competed there in 1952. The Paralympic Summer Games were held abroad in 1960 in Rome and have since taken place subsequently in Perth, Tokyo, Israel, Germany, Toronto, Arnhem, New York, Seoul, Barcelona, Atlanta and Sydney. Sweden hosted the first Paralympic Winter Games in 1976. By the year 2000, athletes from 123 countries competed in Sydney. Just as with other sporting movements, facilities alone were not enough; there had to be professional organization. The

Paralympic Games have attracted large crowds. In 1964 in Tokyo there were 100,000 spectators during the four days of competition. In Beijing 3900 athletes participated.

THE DECLINE OF GERMAN MEDICINE UNDER THE NAZIS

German medicine maintained its pre-eminent status until 1933 but after the advent of Hitler there was a dramatic decline in German medicine and the knowledge was lost. Specialisation and specialist hospitals were opposed in favour of general practice. Anyone who did not remain fit and healthy and contribute to the good of the state became a burden on society, ‘life unworthy of life’, and therefore, the rehabilitation of spinal injury patients was anathema. Under the Nazi regime, unable to practise and fearing for his life and that of his family, Guttmann like many other Jewish doctors fled the country with the aid of the Council for the Assistance of Refugee Academics (CARA).

CONCLUSION

Ludwig Guttmann did not wake up one morning and decide to treat patients with spinal injuries. He was thoroughly trained in Germany in neurology, neurosurgery, research techniques and rehabilitation of patients with peripheral nerve injuries by the world’s finest neurologist Otfrid Foerster. He would have remained in Germany but for the event of the Nazis who forced him to flee his country and seek refuge in the UK. His training and qualifications were not recognised and he was forced to carry out research for 5 years. He was most unhappy and frustrated and wished to abandon research and become a general practitioner until his abilities were recognised by Riddoch and he was offered the thankless task of looking after patients with chronic spinal injuries at Stoke Mandeville Hospital. He adapted and applied existing methods of treatment and instigated new ones that he had been taught in Germany to the treatment of patients with the complications of pressure sores, contractures and urinary infections. Later he realised that the solution to the problem was to treat the patients immediately after injury before the complications had occurred, a treatment pioneered in Sheffield by Frank

Holdsworth (1904-1969). He seized his opportunity with both hands, applying his energy and skill and drive and inspiring leadership. It has to be acknowledged that he came with a huge amount of knowledge and skills that he could adapt and apply to the existing problems achieving a complete fabric of treatment with great success. He acknowledged this saying that other people might have done parts of the treatment but not the whole thing.

> If I have seen further it is by standing on the shoulders of giants
> Sir Isaac Newton (1676)

References

The full references to this chapter can be obtained from Dr. John Silver's book The history of the treatment of spinal injuries, Kluwer Academic/Plenum Publishers New York 2003.

In: Paraplegia
Editor: Agnes A. Holloway
ISBN: 978-1-63482-465-1

Chapter 2

PEDIATRIC SPINAL CORD INJURY

Jeffrey Knox, MD*, Matthew Cage, DO, and Justin Ernat, MD
Tripler Army Medical Center, Honolulu, HI, US

ABSTRACT

Spinal cord injury in the pediatric population is a relatively uncommon but devastating injury. Such injuries in this age group demonstrate numerous significant differences from such injuries in adults. Such differences include patterns and causes of injury, treatment algorithms, and rehabilitation potential. These carry significant implications for evaluation, treatment, and rehabilitation of these patients. In this chapter we review the causes and patterns of injury as well as an overview of treatment and outcomes in this population.

INTRODUCTION

Children represent a unique subgroup of spinal cord injury patients with significant differences in mechanisms, injury patterns, outcomes, and treatment considerations. Understanding these differences is important in managing these complicated patients. Unfortunately, the research on this topic

* Corresponding Author: Jeffrey Knox, MCHK-DSO, 1 Jarrett White Road, Tripler Army Medical Center, Honolulu, HI 96859, Pediatric Spinal Cord Injury Abstract

is relatively sparse and inconsistent with few large multi center studies to help guide understanding of this condition.

The developing spine has many anatomical and biomechanical differences from the adult spine which carry significant implications in pediatric spine trauma [1-3]. While a complete discussion is beyond the scope of the article, important variables include: increased flexibility, small stature, higher head to body ratio, incomplete ossification, and altered facet joint orientation. Ultimately, these changes dissipate and the pediatric spine becomes anatomically similar to that of an adult somewhere between the ages of 8 to 10 years. When considering both these anatomical changes as well as significant developmental and behavioral changes, it becomes clear that children do not represent one single distinct group but rather numerous small subgroups each with unique considerations in evaluation and management of their injuries.

In this chapter we will discuss the pertinent epidemiology, injury characteristics, and outcomes of spinal cord injury in this challenging group of patients.

Epidemiology

Incidence

Spinal cord injury rates are much lower in the pediatric population compared to adults with pediatric injuries comprising only between <4% and 14% of all spinal cord injuries in the United States [4, 5].

Kokosa et al. [6] demonstrated an incidence rate of 18.1 cases per million children per year with a total rate of 1300 cases per year in the United States. Vitale et al. performed an evaluation of a nationwide pediatric inpatient database, which revealed similar incidence data with an incidence of 1.99 cases per 100,000 children and an overall rate of 1455 cases per year. In a Finnish series, Puisto et al. reported a much lower incidence of only 1.9 per 1,000,000 children or 4.3 per 1,000,000 after pre-hospital casualties are included [7].

In comparison, adult spinal cord injury rates range from 25 to 59 cases per million population per year in the United States [8].

While few nation-wide studies have been performed, using a nation-wide database Vitale et al. was able to evaluate regional differences in spinal cord injury incidence rates in the United States.

The highest rates were found in the south where 37.1% of the total cases of pediatric spinal cord injury occurred. This is followed by the midwest and the west with 30.1% and 22.7% respectively. The lowest rates were found in the northeast where only 15.5% of all cases occurred.

AGE

While spinal cord injuries can occur at any age, they become more common with increasing age. Correspondingly, most studies on pediatric spinal cord injury demonstrate the teenage years to be the most prevalent age group.

Vitale et al. evaluated the data from a nationwide database of pediatric hospitalizations and demonstrated an average age at the time of injury to be 14.6 years. Interestingly, this average varies slightly according to gender with females on average younger than males at the time of injury (13.8yrs vs 14.9yrs) [9].

Gender

Numerous studies have demonstrated a significant difference in incidence rates by gender. Similar to the adult population, males sustain spinal cord injuries more frequently than females in general. Incidence rates of spinal cord injury for males range between double [9] and four times [10] the rates in females.

This difference is, however, very age-dependent and is more accentuated in older age groups and the difference diminishes with decreasing age and becomes equivalent in children less than or equal to three years of age [10-12].

Race

There are also significant differences between racial groups. African Americans demonstrate the highest rate of spinal cord injuries and Asian Americans the lowest rate.

At the time of injury, Hispanics tended to be younger on average with an average age of 13.9yrs, and White's tended to be older with an average age of 14.7yrs.

Cause of Injury

The causes of spinal cord injury in children are diverse and vary significantly from those in the adult population. Few large multi center epidemiological studies have been published to give good incidence data on pediatric spinal cord injuries but have yielded similar data on its causes. Motor vehicle crashes represent the most common cause of injury representing 56% [9] of injuries. In the recent series, falls were the second most common cause (14%), followed by gunshot wounds (9%), and sports injuries (8%). In addition to this information for the overall pediatric population, the causes of spinal cord injury are quite variable depending on the age of the children at the time of injury.

Motor vehicle collisions are the most common cause of injury in all age groups, particularly in the younger age groups who tend to have few other high-risk activities. Seatbelt use is an important factor in many of these cases with as many as 67.7% of children who sustained a spinal cord injury not wearing a seatbelt at the time of injury. In addition to non-compliance with restraint use, improper use is common [13] among children and can predispose children to injury, particularly in the thoracolumbar spine [14-18]

In older children and teenagers, sports take on a more important role but variable role. While the rate of spinal cord injury during sports is rare, contact sports, diving, skiing, cycling, and gymnastics are such sports that carry a higher risk [19]. In addition, the rate of spinal cord injury increases with increasing age and ability level as the intensity of the game and skill level advances [20]. Boden et al. reported an annual incidence of 1.10 per 100,000 high school American football players from a nationwide sample. Injuries were over 3x more likely to occur during a game than in practice and most often occurred while making a tackle [21]

The role of violence is an important and often under-appreciated cause of injury in children and is the cause of spinal cord injuries as many as 19% of pre-teens. Surprisingly, firearms were the cause of more than 9% of injuries in a recent nationwide survey [9]. Non-accidental trauma is an important cause of spinal cord injury in very young children, which almost exclusively affects children under the age of three. In this age group, 38% of all spinal trauma in children was found to be secondary to non-accidental trauma in a recent series at a high-volume level 1 pediatric trauma center [22, 23].

Alcohol and drugs are additional factors that are commonly overlooked or under-appreciated in the etiology of pediatric spinal cord injuries. Vitale et al.

reported that they were involved in as many as 30% of such injuries [9] in his series.

Injury Locations

Because of the previously mentioned anatomic differences of the pediatric spine, the location of spinal trauma in children differs significantly from adults and there also is significant variability depending on patient age. The most striking difference is the predominance of cervical spine injuries seen in children as compared to adults. As many as 60-80% of spinal column injuries in children are located in the cervical spine while only 5-34% occur in the thoracolumbar region. [24].

These rates vary significantly depending on the child's age at the time of injury with increasing proportion of cervical spine injuries with decreasing age [24-27]. This difference becomes most distinct in children under the age of three. In this group, 72% of all injuries occur in the cervical spine with upper cervical spine representing the most common location of cervical spine injury [23].

As children mature, the cervical fulcrum shifts distally and the spinal column approaches that of adults resulting in higher rates of middle and lower cervical spine injuries as well as thoracolumbar spine injuries [27-30]. As children age and their spine develops, their injuries resemble that of adults. After the age of 10, thoracolumbar injuries become much more common and represent as much as 70% of patients aged 10-16. [27].

Importantly, children often present with injuries at multiple levels of the spinal column and care should be taken to evaluate for such injuries. Multi-level injuries are found in between 11.8% [31] and 41% [32] and are more common among children between 9 and 16 years of age [33]. Most commonly such injuries are contiguous, being present at adjacent levels in the spinal column, however non-contiguous injuries can occur in between 7% [32] and 37.5% [33].

The recognition of multi-level spinal trauma is crucial in evaluating children with spinal trauma and is often missed during the initial evaluation [31].

Such additional injuries can have significant implications in management of these children and they are also associated with a significantly greater rate of neurologic injury than single-level injuries [31].

Injury Types

In addition to injury location, types of injuries sustained vary significantly based on patient age. In a study by Hofbauer et al. evaluated the patterns of spinal injuries in children and found fracture without subluxation to be the most common and was present in in 64% of patients studied. Fracture with subluxation was found in 21% of patients and subluxation without fracture in 14% of patients [27]. Fractures became more common as patient age increased and subluxations without fracture were more common in younger patients.

In children, the spinal cord typically ends at L3 in the newborn then migrates during childhood to terminate at L1-L2 [34]. Therefore, injuries at or above these levels in the thoracic spine are more likely to cause spinal cord injury than below where the nerve roots are more mobile within the thecal sac [35]. Nerve root injuries are much less common in children compared to adult counterparts but vigiliance for these injuries is still important in evaluating children with spinal trauma.

Cervical Spine Injury

Atlantooccipital (AO) injuries are relatively common and potentially devastating type of cervical spine injury among young children [29]. Such injuries are frequently missed [36, 37], carry a mortality rate of up to 50% and have been found in up to 25% of all fatal pediatric trauma cases. [29, 32, 38]. Because many children die from these injuries prior to arrival at a medical center, their true incidence is often underestimated. Neurologic deficits from injuries at this level can vary including defects of the spinal cord, brain stem, or cranial nerves [37], however up to 80% of such injuries are associated a spinal cord injury [38].

Atlantoaxial (AA) instability injuries without an associated fracture occur less frequently in children than AO injuries, but also occur commonly in younger children. [39].

Fortunately, most such injuries result in minimal neurologic injury [40], however spinal cord injury becomes more common with more severe injuries to this level [41]. In the event that a spinal cord injury does occur with either AA instability or rotatory subluxation, functional status and ventilation requirements are similar to those observed in AO injuries given the cephalad nature of the insult to the cord.

Thoracolumbar Spine Injury

Dogan et al. demonstrated that fractures are the most common type of injury sustained in the thoracolumbar and sacral spine in children, representing 91% of injuries in these locations. Fracture-dislocations occurred in 6.7%, dislocations in 1.1%, and ligamentous injury in 1.1% of patients in the series. At presentation 10.1% had complete spinal cord injuries while 4.5% of patients had incomplete injuries [42]

In burst fractures the middle column of the spine is also disrupted, and thus the contents of the thecal sac are at risk for injury. Retropulsion of the middle column bony fragments can cause direct injury or compression to the neural elements, but it may not always manifest with neurological deficits. Such injuries are relatively uncommon in children compared to adults, representing only 2% of pediatric spinal injuries in a recent series [23]. Vander Have et al. reported a neurologic injury rate of 54% in their series of pediatric burst fractures [35]. Importantly, the risk of spinal cord injury did not correlate with degree of canal compromise, however thoracic fractures were more likely to have spinal cord injury.

Flexion-distraction injuries [43] are rare injuries in the pediatric population, representing only between 4% [32] and 13% [23]. These injuries fail through the anterior and middle columns as a result of a compressive or distractive force and are almost exclusively caused by motor vehicle crashes. In children, L2-L3 is the most common level injured in this fashion [17, 18], however such injuries can occur throughout the thoracolumbar spine. Arkader et al. reported a neurologic injury rate of 43% among children with this injury type with neurologic injury much more common in patients who were unrestrained at the time of injury (42%) than those restrained (10%) [44]. The rate of paraplegia in this injury type ranges from 15% (17) to 23% [17, 43].

High-energy torsional, distraction, or shearing mechanisms can lead to fracture-dislocations of the thoracolumbar spine. Although uncommon, these injuries are highly associated with spinal cord injuries, and thus must be reduced and stabilized to preserve function or prevent neurologic deterioration. [34]

In older children (10-16 years), apophyseal fractures and disc herniations can occur and may result in neurologic deficit or spinal cord injury depending on the level and location. [45, 46]. These injuries are much less common in children and account for only 0.5-6.8% of all the discectomies performed in all ages [47-50]. Separation of the ring apophysis, or fracture, has been reported to occur in 5.7% of all disc herniation patients, but the actual incidence in adolescent patients is not truly known. [51] Chang in 2008 reported on ring apophysis fractures associated with adolescent disc herniation. [45]. They found that these injuries most commonly involve L5-S1 and the upper endplate. Apophyseal fracture was more commonly seen at L5-S1 versus L4-L5 where herniation alone was more common. The neurologic injury rate for such injuries is not well described in the literature.

Spinal Cord Injury Without Radiologic Abnormality (SCIWORA)

Spinal cord injury without radiologic abnormality (SCIWORA) is an injury pattern that is almost exclusively seen in children. The etiology of this injury is thought to be a result of a greater elasticity of the vertebral column whereby the spinal column can tolerate more stretch than the spinal cord. An alternate possible etiology is spinal cord ischemia due to a more tenuous spinal cord blood supply in children [52, 53].

The definition of this injury type continues to evolve with the increasing use of MRI in pediatric spinal trauma. This was described by Pang and Wilberger in 1982 as a patient with signs of myelopathy with no injury or fractures on radiographs or tomograms. [54]. This definition excluded penetrating trauma, electrical shock, obstetric complications, and congenital spine anomalies. With the advent of MRI, many cases that were previously classified as SCIWORA are now known to be caused by isolated ligamentous injuries which were not seen at the time due to the unavailability of MRI. Currently, many consider SCIWORA to be only those injuries with no radiographic anomalies including MRI. Using this more restrictive definition, SCIWORA is a much less common entity than was previously thought.

The incidence of this injury varies significantly based on the age of patients studied as well as the definition used. SCIWORA has been reported to comprise between 19 and 34% of all pediatric spinal cord injuries [55] and between 14 and 66% of pediatric cervical spine injuries [29, 38, 56]. Older studies report SCIWORA to be responsible for greater than 20% of traumatic spinal cord injuries [5, 11, 57, 58] with a review of 14 series involving 617 children presenting with traumatic myelopathy reporting a 36% incidence of SCIWORA [29]. In contrast, a recent study of pediatric spinal trauma utilizing the more restrictive definition of SCIWORA found a rate of less than 3% [23].

SCIWORA in younger children occurs more commonly in the upper cervical spine. [29, 54, 59-61] These injuries are associated with severe neurological deficits and they often present in a delayed fashion [58, 60-64]. 70% of injuries in young children are neurologically complete at the time of presentation [56]. SCIWORA in adolescents, however, is rarely complete and is more often located in the lower cervical and thoracic spine. Lumbar spine SCIWORA has not been described in children.

Outcomes of SCIWORA injuries are variable and strongly associated with the severity of the initial injury [61, 65]. Mild to moderate cord injuries have good potential for functional recovery with reports of regaining full function [65, 66]. Hamilton and Myles showed that 74% of patients with incomplete SCIWORA demonstrated significant improvement with 59% demonstrating a complete recovery of neurologic function [66]. In contrast, recovery rates for complete injuries have been reported as less than 10% [56]. Bosch et al. reported that patients with SCIWORA do not typically deteriorate after their initial recovery [67]. However, recurrence does not preclude the patient from experiencing a full recovery of neurologic function.

ASSOCIATED INJURIES

Spinal trauma in children typically occurs in the setting of high-energy trauma and is commonly associated with multiple other injuries. Head injuries are particularly common in children with spinal trauma, with incidence rates between 37% [3] and 64.3% [27]. Head injuries are more commonly associated with cervical spine injuries, and become more common with more cephalad spine injuries [26, 38, 68, 69]. Osenbach et al. reported that head injuries will occur in 20% concomitantly with spine trauma, however, 66% of these head injuries were in the setting of cervical spine trauma. [26]. Brown et al. in 2001 noted 59/103 patients to have injuries concomitantly with cervical spine trauma. [38] The majority were closed head injuries. Interestingly, 90% of the children who died had concomitant closed head injuries. Younger children wore more likely to experience a closed head injury, as well (72% vs. 45%). Cirak et al. in 2004 [3], found head/brain injuries were the most likely associated injury in the setting of spine trauma occurring concurrently 37% of the time. (3) Despite the association with cervical trauma, head injuries are found in greater than 30% of patients who sustain thoracolumbar spine injuries [43].

Thoracic and intra-abdominal injuries are also common concomitant injuries in children with spinal trauma [27, 43] and occur more commonly in older children between 10 and 17 years of age [27]. Such injuries are particularly associated with thoracolumbar spine injuries, particularly flexion distraction injuries which are associated with thoraco-abdominal injuries in up to 42% of patients [43]. Common associated injuries with thoracic or thoracolumbar spinal trauma include small bowel injuries, pancreatic rupture, hemothorax or pneumothorax, lung contusions, and aortic injury. [34]. In Osenbach's series 8% of patients had intraabdominal injuries and 4% presented with blunt thoracic injuries. [26]. Long bone fractures were also present in 8% of patients. In a study by Hofbauer et al. on pediatric polytrauma patients with spine injuries, [27], the most common associated non-spinal injuries were thoracic (89.3%), followed by traumatic brain injuries (64.3%). Abdominal injuries were also common (57%) and tended to occur in older patients between 10 and 17 years of age.

OUTCOMES

Neurologic Recovery

Despite higher rates of complete spinal cord injury, clinical evidence would suggest that children have a higher capacity for neurologic recovery after SCI [70-73]. In the animal model numerous mechanisms have been described that provide insight into the biologic processes that occur in the immature spinal cord after injury. In a landmark study by Kalil et al., infant hamsters were shown to have massive regrowth of their severed axons via new brainstem pathways to the correct terminal sites [74]. This was the first study of its kind to demonstrate the regenerative potential in the infant mammalian central nervous system. Experimental data on neonatal cats has shown the formation of aberrant corticospinal pathways and retrograde degeneration of brainstem-spinal pathways after spinal cord damage, neither of which occur in adult cats [75]. Collectively, the work done in histologic and clinical animal studies demonstrates a regenerative potential of the immature spinal cord that is not present in adults. Additionally, there may be factors present in adult spinal cord injury patients that may inhibit the regenerative potential of the central nervous system. It is widely believe that the comorbidities typically seen in adult patients, such as diabetes and hypertension, inhibit the adult patient's ability to recover from SCI [76].

As in adult patients, complete injuries in pediatric patients carry a worse prognosis than incomplete injuries. Complete injuries are also more likely to be associated with certain long term complications such as; autonomic dysreflexia, severe scoliosis, hip dysplasia, pressure ulcers and bowel and bladder dysfunction [76]. However substantial neurologic recovery and even independent ambulation can often been seen after complete pediatric SCI [70]. In their series of 20 pediatric patients with complete SCI, Wang et al. demonstrated that of the 13 patients who survived their injury, six (46%) demonstrated significant functional improvement and 5 of those patients eventually became ambulatory [70]. In contrast to adults who have little recovery potential beyond the acute post injury period [77, 78], pediatric patients have demonstrated meaningful neurologic improvement for up to one year after injury [70].

Factors associated with increased likelihood of neurologic recovery include younger age, incomplete neurologic injury, and SCIWORA [70]. Prognosis for neurologic recovery is best predicted by their presenting neurologic status [71, 79].

MRI findings have also been correlated with neurologic recovery. Grabb et al. evaluated the MRI findings in spinal cord injury and found that major cord hemorrhage involving most of the transverse area of the cord and cord discontinuity were associated with complete neurologic injuries. Edema without evidence of hemorrhage or minor cord hemorrhage involving less than 50% of the transverse area of the cord were associated with incomplete neurologic recovery with residual deficits. Normal MR imaging of the spinal cord without signal abnormality or contour distortion was associated with complete neurological recovery independent of the presenting neurological syndrome. Davis et al. demonstrated that both hemorrhagic and nonhemorrhagic lesions on MRI could be associated with significant, persistent cord deficits. [80].

Role of Steroids

High dose corticosteroid use in the setting of spinal cord injury is a controversial but widely used treatment in an attempt to minimize further neurologic injury and improve neurologic outcomes. Despite early enthusiasm for its use, the use of steroids has become increasingly controversial and has largely fallen out of favor due to concerns over potential complications of the treatment with limited potential benefit [81]. Although numerous studies have been published on this treatment in adults, nearly all papers published have eliminated pediatric patients from analysis. As such, there is no published evidence that supports improved neurologic outcome and administration of steroids following pediatric spinal cord injury [71]. Despite the lack of evidence for improved neurologic outcome with steroid treatment, its use is commonplace. Recent studies have demonstrated that the high rate of complications from steroid treatment seen in adult patients is not seen in the pediatric patient [82, 83].

Role of Surgical Intervention

Due to limited available data, the principles of treatment for pediatric spinal cord injury have been extrapolated from adult data. Those treatment principles include; rapid stabilization, rigid orthotic treatment, and when necessary, surgical decompression and instrumentation. The use of instrumentation to treat pediatric spinal column fractures has traditionally been controversial. There is a lack of evidence in the pediatric literature for outcomes following decompression and instrumented stabilization. Most of the current studies are retrospective, and combine the outcomes of both non-operative and operatively treated children [30, 42, 84-86]. The primary indication for the use of instrumentation in an injured pediatric spine is instability. The recent development of smaller pedicle screws has facilitated the operative stabilization of unstable cervical spine fractures in pediatric patients [24].

Complications

As in the adult population, the complications of SCI are numerous and include urinary dysfunction, spasticity, pain syndromes, psychological sequelae, respiratory insufficiency, scoliosis and hip dysplasia [76].

Autonomic Dysreflexia

Autonomic dysreflexia (AD) is a potentially life-threatening condition in which overstimulation of the autonomic nervous system following spinal cord injury leads to paroxysmal hypertension, bradycardia, profuse sweating, and sometimes cognitive impairment. Treatment of autonomic dysreflexia involved administration of anti-hypertensives and removing the triggering stimuli, often times fecal impaction, bladder distention or urinary tract infection. Schottler et al. demonstrated 34% of children with a SCI at or above the level T6 experienced autonomic dysreflexia at a median duration of 8 years and 10 months after injury [87]. Those with complete lesions were more likely to experience autonomic dysreflexia compared to those within complete lesions.

Scoliosis

Children who sustain a SCI are at a substantial risk of developing scoliosis later in life. The deformity is believed to be the result of a paraspinal muscle imbalance resulting from the spinal cord injury with other potential etiologies such as wheelchair dependence, and hip flexion contractures [24, 88-90]. The age that the patient sustained a spinal cord injury carries significant importance in the risk of developing scoliosis with a rate approaching 100% if the injury occurs prior to the patient's growth spurt [91]. In a series of patients under the age of 5 who had sustained a spinal cord injury, Schottler et al., demonstrated almost all (96%) developed scoliosis, with more than half (63%) developing a curve of greater than 40 degrees at an average follow up of 10.8 years [87]. Gender and level of injury was found not to be significant factors in predicting the development of scoliosis, however those with complete injuries and younger patients were much more likely to develop larger curves [87, 90].

Because of the frequency of this complication, children who have sustained a spinal cord injury should be closely followed until skeletal maturity. Once a deformity has been identified, early intervention is recommended. It has been recommended that brace treatment should be implemented before the curve reaches 10 degrees to prevent scoliosis progression. Curves less than 20 degrees should be braced to delay surgical correction [92]. When bracing fails to control curve progression, surgical intervention is often necessary in a manner similar to the treatment of neuromuscular scoliosis [71]. The rate of surgery for the development of scoliosis following spinal cord injury varies and ranges from 45%-77% [91-93].

Hip Dysplasia

Hip pathology including dysplasia, dislocation and flexion contracture are common sequelae of pediatric SCI. In Schottler's series of pediatric patients with SCI under the age of 5, 57% of the 146 participants with greater than 1 year of follow up demonstrated hip dysplasia. Despite the relative frequency, only 8% had required surgery for their hip pathology during the study period. Paraplegia (X2 – 4.67) and complete neurologic injury (X2 = 9.53) were more significantly associated with the development of hip complications [87].

Conclusion

Children represent a unique group of patients in spinal cord injury. The developing spine contains significant anatomic and biomechanical differences from the mature spine, which bears important implications in the location and type of spinal trauma that children sustain. SCIWORA represents an important type of injury within this population that carries unique prognostic and diagnostic implications. Additionally, it remains important to recognize that children have a higher innate potential for improvement after spinal cord injury compared to adults with comparable injuries. Children who sustain a spinal cord injury are subjected to a longer lifetime with this deficit compared to adults and therefore have a large potential to develop complications during their lifetime. While these complications are generally the same as those in adults, children have a high rate of scoliosis as well as hip dysplasia which are not seen as commonly among adults.

References

[1] Slotkin JR, Lu Y, Wood KB. Thoracolumbar spinal trauma in children. *Neurosurg. Clin. N. Am.* 2007;18(4):621-30. doi: 10.1016/j.nec. 2007.07.003. PubMed PMID: 17991587.

[2] d'Amato C. Pediatric spinal trauma: injuries in very young children. *Clin. Orthop. Relat. Res.* 2005(432):34-40. PubMed PMID: 15738801.

[3] Cirak B, Ziegfeld S, Knight VM, Chang D, Avellino AM, Paidas CN. Spinal injuries in children. *J. Pediatr. Surg.* 2004;39(4):607-12. PubMed PMID: 15065038.

[4] Gehrig R, Michaelis LS. Statistics of acute paraplegia and tetraplegia on a national scale. Switzerland 1960-67. *Paraplegia*. 1968;6(2):93-5. doi: 10.1038/sc.1968.16. PubMed PMID: 5683734.

[5] Kewalramani LS, Kraus JF, Sterling HM. Acute spinal-cord lesions in a pediatric population: epidemiological and clinical features. *Paraplegia*. 1980;18(3):206-19. doi: 10.1038/sc.1980.36. PubMed PMID: 7413243.

[6] Kokoska ER, Keller MS, Rallo MC, Weber TR. Characteristics of pediatric cervical spine injuries. *J. Pediatr. Surg*. 2001;36(1):100-5. doi: 10.1053/jpsu.2001.20022. PubMed PMID: 11150446.

[7] Puisto V, Kääriäinen S, Impinen A, Parkkila T, Vartiainen E, Jalanko T, et al. Incidence of spinal and spinal cord injuries and their surgical treatment in children and adolescents: a population-based study. *Spine* (Phila Pa 1976). 2010;35(1):104-7. doi: 10.1097/BRS.0b013e3181c64423. PubMed PMID: 20042961.

[8] Devivo MJ. Epidemiology of traumatic spinal cord injury: trends and future implications. *Spinal. Cord*. 2012;50(5):365-72. doi: 10.1038/sc.2011.178. PubMed PMID: 22270188.

[9] Vitale MG, Goss JM, Matsumoto H, Roye DP. Epidemiology of pediatric spinal cord injury in the United States: years 1997 and 2000. *J Pediatr Orthop*. 2006;26(6):745-9. doi: 10.1097/01.bpo.0000235400.49536.83. PubMed PMID: 17065938.

[10] DeVivo MJ, Vogel LC. Epidemiology of spinal cord injury in children and adolescents. *J. Spinal. Cord. Med*. 2004;27 Suppl 1:S4-10. PubMed PMID: 15503696.

[11] Ruge JR, Sinson GP, McLone DG, Cerullo LJ. Pediatric spinal injury: the very young. *J. Neurosurg*. 1988;68(1):25-30. doi: 10.3171/jns.1988.68.1.0025. PubMed PMID: 3335908.

[12] Bilston LE, Brown J. Pediatric spinal injury type and severity are age and mechanism dependent. *Spine* (Phila Pa 1976). 2007;32(21):2339-47. doi: 10.1097/BRS.0b013e3181558886. PubMed PMID: 17906576.

[13] Greenspan AI, Dellinger AM, Chen J. Restraint use and seating position among children less than 13 years of age: Is it still a problem? *J. Safety Res*. 2010;41(2):183-5. doi: 10.1016/j.jsr.2010.03.001. PubMed PMID: 20497804.

[14] Papavasiliou A, Stanton J, Sinha P, Forder J, Skyrme A. The complexity of seat belt injuries including spinal injury in the pediatric population: a case report of a 6-year-old boy and the literature review. *Eur. J. Emerg*. Med. 2007;14(3):180-3. doi: 10.1097/MEJ.0b013e32801430e2. PubMed PMID: 17473618.

[15] Lane JC. The seat belt syndrome in children. *Accid. Anal. Prev.* 1994;26(6):813-20. PubMed PMID: 7857496.

[16] Valent F, McGwin G, Hardin W, Johnston C, Rue LW. Restraint use and injury patterns among children involved in motor vehicle collisions. *J. Trauma.* 2002;52(4):745-51. PubMed PMID: 11956394.

[17] Rumball K, Jarvis J. Seat-belt injuries of the spine in young children. *J. Bone Joint Surg. Br.* 1992;74(4):571-4. PubMed PMID: 1624518.

[18] Glassman SD, Johnson JR, Holt RT. Seatbelt injuries in children. *J. Trauma.* 1992;33(6):882-6. PubMed PMID: 1474632.

[19] Maxfield BA. Sports-related injury of the pediatric spine. *Radiol. Clin. North Am.* 2010;48(6):1237-48. doi: 10.1016/j.rcl.2010.07.006. PubMed PMID: 21094408.

[20] Caine D, Caine C, Maffulli N. Incidence and distribution of pediatric sport-related injuries. *Clin. J. Sport Med.* 2006;16(6):500-13. doi: 10.1097/01.jsm.0000251181.36582.a0. PubMed PMID: 17119363.

[21] Boden BP, Tacchetti RL, Cantu RC, Knowles SB, Mueller FO. Catastrophic cervical spine injuries in high school and college football players. *Am. J. Sports Med.* 2006;34(8):1223-32. doi: 10.1177/0363546506288306. PubMed PMID: 16816152.

[22] Knox J, Schneider J, Wimberly RL, Riccio AI. Characteristics of spinal injuries secondary to nonaccidental trauma. *J. Pediatr. Orthop.* 2014;34(4):376-81. doi: 10.1097/BPO.0000000000000111. PubMed PMID: 24172665.

[23] Knox JB, Schneider JE, Cage JM, Wimberly RL, Riccio AI. Spine trauma in very young children: a retrospective study of 206 patients presenting to a level 1 pediatric trauma center. *J. Pediatr. Orthop.* 2014;34(7):698-702. doi: 10.1097/BPO.0000000000000167. PubMed PMID: 25207594.

[24] Parent S, Dimar J, Dekutoski M, Roy-Beaudry M. Unique features of pediatric spinal cord injury. *Spine* (Phila Pa 1976). 2010;35(21 Suppl):S202-8. doi: 10.1097/BRS.0b013e3181f35acb. PubMed PMID: 20881463.

[25] Reilly CW. Pediatric spine trauma. *J Bone Joint Surg Am.* 2007;89 Suppl 1:98-107. doi: 10.2106/JBJS.F.00244. PubMed PMID: 17272427.

[26] Osenbach RK, Menezes AH. Pediatric spinal cord and vertebral column injury. *Neurosurgery.* 1992;30(3):385-90. PubMed PMID: 1620302.

[27] Hofbauer M, Jaindl M, Höchtl LL, Ostermann RC, Kdolsky R, Aldrian S. Spine injuries in polytraumatized pediatric patients: characteristics and experience from a Level I trauma center over two decades. *J.*

Trauma Acute. Care Surg. 2012;73(1):156-61. doi: 10.1097/TA.0b013e31824e32b5. PubMed PMID: 22743385.

[28] Apple DF, Anson CA, Hunter JD, Bell RB. Spinal cord injury in youth. *Clin. Pediatr.* (Phila). 1995;34(2):90-5. PubMed PMID: 7729113.

[29] McCall T, Fassett D, Brockmeyer D. Cervical spine trauma in children: a review. *Neurosurg Focus.* 2006;20(2):E5. PubMed PMID: 16512656.

[30] Dogan S, Safavi-Abbasi S, Theodore N, Horn E, Rekate HL, Sonntag VK. Pediatric subaxial cervical spine injuries: origins, management, and outcome in 51 patients. *Neurosurg. Focus.* 2006;20(2):E1. doi: 10.3171/foc.2006.20.2.2. PubMed PMID: 16512652.

[31] Firth GB, Kingwell SP, Moroz PJ. Pediatric noncontiguous spinal injuries: the 15-year experience at a level 1 trauma center. Spine (Phila Pa 1976). 2012;37(10):E599-608. doi: 10.1097/BRS.0b013e31824079ea. PubMed PMID: 22544284.

[32] Carreon LY, Glassman SD, Campbell MJ. Pediatric spine fractures: a review of 137 hospital admissions. *J. Spinal Disord. Tech.* 2004;17(6):477-82. PubMed PMID: 15570118.

[33] Mortazavi MM, Dogan S, Civelek E, Tubbs RS, Theodore N, Rekate HL, et al. Pediatric multilevel spine injuries: an institutional experience. *Childs Nerv Syst.* 2011;27(7):1095-100. doi: 10.1007/s00381-010-1348-y. PubMed PMID: 21110031.

[34] Daniels AH, Sobel AD, Eberson CP. Pediatric thoracolumbar spine trauma. *J. Am. Acad. Orthop. Surg.* 2013;21(12):707-16. doi: 10.5435/JAAOS-21-12-707. PubMed PMID: 24292927.

[35] Vander Have KL, Caird MS, Gross S, Farley FA, Graziano GA, Stauff M, et al. Burst fractures of the thoracic and lumbar spine in children and adolescents. *J. Pediatr. Orthop.* 2009;29(7):713-9. doi: 10.1097/BPO.0b013e3181b76a44. PubMed PMID: 20104151.

[36] Sun PP, Poffenbarger GJ, Durham S, Zimmerman RA. Spectrum of occipitoatlantoaxial injury in young children. *J. Neurosurg.* 2000;93(1 Suppl):28-39. PubMed PMID: 10879755.

[37] Steinmetz MP, Lechner RM, Anderson JS. Atlantooccipital dislocation in children: presentation, diagnosis, and management. *Neurosurg. Focus.* 2003;14(2):ecp1. PubMed PMID: 15727431.

[38] Brown RL, Brunn MA, Garcia VF. Cervical spine injuries in children: a review of 103 patients treated consecutively at a level 1 pediatric trauma center. *J. Pediatr. Surg.* 2001;36(8):1107-14. doi: 10.1053/jpsu.2001.25665. PubMed PMID: 11479837.

[39] McGrory BJ, Klassen RA, Chao EY, Staeheli JW, Weaver AL. Acute fractures and dislocations of the cervical spine in children and adolescents. *J. Bone Joint. Surg. Am.* 1993;75(7):988-95. PubMed PMID: 8335674.

[40] Wong DA, Mack RP, Craigmile TK. Traumatic atlantoaxial dislocation without fracture of the odontoid. *Spine* (Phila Pa 1976). 1991;16(5):587-9. PubMed PMID: 2053005.

[41] Phillips WA, Hensinger RN. The management of rotatory atlanto-axial subluxation in children. *J. Bone Joint Surg. Am.* 1989;71(5):664-8. PubMed PMID: 2732254.

[42] Dogan S, Safavi-Abbasi S, Theodore N, Chang SW, Horn EM, Mariwalla NR, et al. Thoracolumbar and sacral spinal injuries in children and adolescents: a review of 89 cases. *J. Neurosurg.* 2007;106(6 Suppl):426-33. doi: 10.3171/ped.2007.106.6.426. PubMed PMID: 17566397.

[43] Louman-Gardiner K, Mulpuri K, Perdios A, Tredwell S, Cripton PA. Pediatric lumbar Chance fractures in British Columbia: chart review and analysis of the use of shoulder restraints in MVAs. Accid Anal Prev. 2008;40(4):1424-9. doi: 10.1016/j.aap.2008.03.007. PubMed PMID: 18606276.

[44] Arkader A, Warner WC, Tolo VT, Sponseller PD, Skaggs DL. Pediatric Chance fractures: a multicenter perspective. *J. Pediatr. Orthop.* 2011;31(7):741-4. doi: 10.1097/BPO.0b013e31822f1b0b. PubMed PMID:21926870.

[45] Chang CH, Lee ZL, Chen WJ, Tan CF, Chen LH. Clinical significance of ring apophysis fracture in adolescent lumbar disc herniation. *Spine* (Phila Pa 1976). 2008;33(16):1750-4. doi: 10.1097/ BRS.0b013e31817d1d12. PubMed PMID: 18628708.

[46] Shirado O, Yamazaki Y, Takeda N, Minami A. Lumbar disc herniation associated with separation of the ring apophysis: is removal of the detached apophyses mandatory to achieve satisfactory results? *Clin. Orthop. Relat Res.* 2005(431):120-8. PubMed PMID: 15685064.

[47] DeOrio JK, Bianco AJ. Lumbar disc excision in children and adolescents. J. Bone Joint. Surg. Am. 1982;64(7):991-6. PubMed PMID: 6214560.

[48] Epstein JA, Epstein NE, Marc J, Rosenthal AD, Lavine LS. Lumbar intervertebral disk herniation in teenage children: recognition and management of associated anomalies. *Spine* (Phila Pa 1976). 1984;9(4):427-32. PubMed PMID: 6474257.

[49] Ishihara H, Matsui H, Hirano N, Tsuji H. Lumbar intervertebral disc herniation in children less than 16 years of age. Long-term follow-up study of surgically managed cases. *Spine* (Phila Pa 1976). 1997;22(17):2044-9. PubMed PMID: 9306537.
[50] Rugtveit A. Juvenile lumbar disc herniations. Acta Orthop Scand. 1966;37(4):348-56. PubMed PMID: 5961764.
[51] Yang IK, Bahk YW, Choi KH, Paik MW, Shinn KS. Posterior lumbar apophyseal ring fractures: a report of 20 cases. *Neuroradiology*. 1994;36(6):453-5. PubMed PMID: 7991090.
[52] Choi JU, Hoffman HJ, Hendrick EB, Humphreys RP, Keith WS. Traumatic infarction of the spinal cord in children. *J. Neurosurg*. 1986;65(5):608-10. doi: 10.3171/jns.1986.65.5.0608. PubMed PMID: 3772446.
[53] LEVENTHAL HR. Birth injuries of the spinal cord. *J. Pediatr.* 1960;56:447-53. PubMed PMID: 14416159.
[54] Pang D, Wilberger JE. Spinal cord injury without radiographic abnormalities in children. *J Neurosurg*. 1982;57(1):114-29. doi: 10.3171/jns.1982.57.1.0114. PubMed PMID: 7086488.
[55] Launay F, Leet AI, Sponseller PD. Pediatric spinal cord injury without radiographic abnormality: a meta-analysis. *Clin. Orthop. Relat. Res.* 2005(433):166-70. PubMed PMID: 15805953.
[56] Dickman CA, Zabramski JM, Hadley MN, Rekate HL, Sonntag VK. Pediatric spinal cord injury without radiographic abnormalities: report of 26 cases and review of the literature. *J. Spinal Disord.* 1991;4(3):296-305. PubMed PMID: 1802160.
[57] Burke DC. Traumatic spinal paralysis in children. *Paraplegia.* 1974;11(4):268-76. doi: 10.1038/sc.1973.39. PubMed PMID: 4827225.
[58] Hadley MN, Zabramski JM, Browner CM, Rekate H, Sonntag VK. Pediatric spinal trauma. Review of 122 cases of spinal cord and vertebral column injuries. *J. Neurosurg*. 1988;68(1):18-24. doi: 10.3171/jns.1988.68.1.0018. PubMed PMID: 3335907.
[59] Grabb PA, Pang D. Magnetic resonance imaging in the evaluation of spinal cord injury without radiographic abnormality in children. *Neurosurgery*. 1994;35(3):406-14; discussion 14. PubMed PMID: 7800131.
[60] Osenbach RK, Menezes AH. Spinal cord injury without radiographic abnormality in children. *Pediatr. Neurosci.* 1989;15(4):168-74; discussion 75. PubMed PMID: 2485911.

[61] Pang D, Pollack IF. Spinal cord injury without radiographic abnormality in children--the SCIWORA syndrome. *J. Trauma*. 1989;29(5):654-64. PubMed PMID: 2724383.
[62] Walsh JW, Stevens DB, Young AB. Traumatic paraplegia in children without contiguous spinal fracture or dislocation. *Neurosurgery*. 1983;12(4):439-45. PubMed PMID: 6856070.
[63] Yngve DA, Harris WP, Herndon WA, Sullivan JA, Gross RH. Spinal cord injury without osseous spine fracture. *J. Pediatr. Orthop*. 1988;8(2):153-9. PubMed PMID: 3350948.
[64] Ahmann PA, Smith SA, Schwartz JF, Clark DB. Spinal cord infarction due to minor trauma in children. *Neurology*. 1975;25(4):301-7. PubMed PMID: 1168316.
[65] Pang D. Spinal cord injury without radiographic abnormality in children, 2 decades later. *Neurosurgery*. 2004;55(6):1325-42; discussion 42-3. PubMed PMID: 15574214.
[66] Hamilton MG, Myles ST. Pediatric spinal injury: review of 61 deaths. *J. Neurosurg*. 1992;77(5):705-8. doi: 10.3171/jns.1992.77.5.0705. PubMed PMID: 1403111.
[67] Bosch PP, Vogt MT, Ward WT. Pediatric spinal cord injury without radiographic abnormality (SCIWORA): the absence of occult instability and lack of indication for bracing. *Spine* (Phila Pa 1976). 2002;27(24):2788-800. doi: 10.1097/01.BRS.0000035687.53040.F5. PubMed PMID: 12486348.
[68] Nitecki S, Moir CR. Predictive factors of the outcome of traumatic cervical spine fracture in children. *J. Pediatr. Surg*. 1994;29(11):1409-11. PubMed PMID: 7844708.
[69] Jones TM, Anderson PA, Noonan KJ. Pediatric cervical spine trauma. J Am Acad Orthop Surg. 2011;19(10):600-11. PubMed PMID: 21980025.
[70] Wang MY, Hoh DJ, Leary SP, Griffith P, McComb JG. High rates of neurological improvement following severe traumatic pediatric spinal cord injury. *Spine* (Phila Pa 1976). 2004;29(13):1493-7; discussion E266. PubMed PMID: 15223946.
[71] Parent S, Mac-Thiong JM, Roy-Beaudry M, Sosa JF, Labelle H. Spinal cord injury in the pediatric population: a systematic review of the literature. *J. Neurotrauma*. 2011;28(8):1515-24. doi: 10.1089/neu.2009.1153. PubMed PMID: 21501096; PubMed Central PMCID: PMCPMC3143390.

[72] Birney TJ, Hanley EN. Traumatic cervical spine injuries in childhood and adolescence. *Spine* (Phila Pa 1976). 1989;14(12):1277-82. PubMed PMID: 2617355.

[73] Dickman CA, Rekate HL, Sonntag VK, Zabramski JM. Pediatric spinal trauma: vertebral column and spinal cord injuries in children. Pediatr *Neurosci.* 1989;15(5):237-55; discussion 56. PubMed PMID: 2488952.

[74] Kalil K, Reh T. Regrowth of severed axons in the neonatal central nervous system: establishment of normal connections. Science. 1979;205(4411):1158-61. PubMed PMID: 472734.

[75] Bregman BS, Goldberger ME. Anatomical plasticity and sparing of function after spinal cord damage in neonatal cats. *Science.* 1982;217(4559):553-5. PubMed PMID: 7089581.

[76] Sharpe AN, Forsyth R. Acute paediatric paraplegia: a case series review. *Eur. J. Paediatr. Neurol.* 2013;17(6):620-4. doi: 10.1016/j.ejpn. 2013.05.014. PubMed PMID: 23806995.

[77] Fawcett JW, Curt A, Steeves JD, Coleman WP, Tuszynski MH, Lammertse D, et al. Guidelines for the conduct of clinical trials for spinal cord injury as developed by the ICCP panel: spontaneous recovery after spinal cord injury and statistical power needed for therapeutic clinical trials. Spinal Cord. 2007;45(3):190-205. doi: 10.1038/sj.sc.3102007. PubMed PMID: 17179973.

[78] Marino RJ, Ditunno JF, Donovan WH, Maynard F. Neurologic recovery after traumatic spinal cord injury: data from the Model Spinal Cord Injury Systems. *Arch. Phys. Med. Rehabil.* 1999;80(11):1391-6. PubMed PMID: 10569432.

[79] Chien LC, Wu JC, Chen YC, Liu L, Huang WC, Chen TJ, et al. Age, sex, and socio-economic status affect the incidence of pediatric spinal cord injury: an eleven-year national cohort study. PLoS One. 2012;7(6):e39264. doi: 10.1371/journal.pone.0039264. PubMed PMID: 22761749; PubMed Central PMCID: PMCPMC3382245.

[80] Davis PC, Reisner A, Hudgins PA, Davis WE, O'Brien MS. Spinal injuries in children: role of MR. AJNR *Am. J. Neuroradiol.* 1993;14(3):607-17. PubMed PMID: 8517348.

[81] Ito Y, Sugimoto Y, Tomioka M, Kai N, Tanaka M. Does high dose methylprednisolone sodium succinate really improve neurological status in patient with acute cervical cord injury?: a prospective study about neurological recovery and early complications. *Spine* (Phila Pa 1976). 2009;34(20):2121-4. doi: 10.1097/BRS.0b013e3181b613c7. PubMed PMID: 19713878.

[82] Cage CP, Knox MJ, Wimberly RL, Shaha S, Jo C, Riccio AI. Complications Associated With High-dose Corticosteroid Administration in Children With Spinal Cord Injury. *J. Pediatr. Orthop.* 2014. doi: 10.1097/BPO.0000000000000364. PubMed PMID: 25494031.

[83] Arora B, Suresh S. Spinal cord injuries in older children: is there a role for high-dose methylprednisolone? *Pediatr Emerg Care.* 2011;27(12):1192-4. doi: 10.1097/PEC.0b013e31823b4d06. PubMed PMID: 22158284.

[84] Haque A, Price AV, Sklar FH, Swift DM, Weprin BE, Sacco DJ. Screw fixation of the upper cervical spine in the pediatric population. Clinical article. *J. Neurosurg. Pediatr.* 2009;3(6):529-33. doi: 10.3171/2009.2.PEDS08149. PubMed PMID: 19485741.

[85] Crostelli M, Mariani M, Mazza O, Ascani E. Cervical fixation in the pediatric patient: our experience. *Eur. Spine J.* 2009;18 Suppl 1:20-8. doi: 10.1007/s00586-009-0980-2. PubMed PMID: 19404690; PubMed Central PMCID: PMCPMC2899601.

[86] Chamoun RB, Relyea KM, Johnson KK, Whitehead WE, Curry DJ, Luerssen TG, et al. Use of axial and subaxial translaminar screw fixation in the management of upper cervical spinal instability in a series of 7 children. *Neurosurgery.* 2009;64(4):734-9; discussion 9. doi: 10.1227/01.NEU.0000338950.46195.9C. PubMed PMID: 19349831.

[87] Schottler J, Vogel LC, Sturm P. Spinal cord injuries in young children: a review of children injured at 5 years of age and younger. *Dev. Med. Child* Neurol. 2012;54(12):1138-43. doi: 10.1111/j.1469-8749.2012.04411.x. PubMed PMID: 22998495.

[88] Bergström EM, Henderson NJ, Short DJ, Frankel HL, Jones PR. The relation of thoracic and lumbar fracture configuration to the development of late deformity in childhood spinal cord injury. *Spine* (Phila Pa 1976). 2003;28(2):171-6. doi: 10.1097/01.BRS. 0000041575. 64140.4A. PubMed PMID: 12544935.

[89] Bergström EM, Short DJ, Frankel HL, Henderson NJ, Jones PR. The effect of childhood spinal cord injury on skeletal development: a retrospective study. *Spinal Cord.* 1999;37(12):838-46. PubMed PMID: 10602526.

[90] Lancourt JE, Dickson JH, Carter RE. Paralytic spinal deformity following traumatic spinal-cord injury in children and adolescents. *J. Bone Joint. Surg. Am.* 1981;63(1):47-53. PubMed PMID: 7451526.

[91] Dearolf WW, Betz RR, Vogel LC, Levin J, Clancy M, Steel HH. Scoliosis in pediatric spinal cord-injured patients. *J. Pediatr. Orthop.* 1990;10(2):214-8. PubMed PMID: 2312704.

[92] Mehta S, Betz RR, Mulcahey MJ, McDonald C, Vogel LC, Anderson C. Effect of bracing on paralytic scoliosis secondary to spinal cord injury. *J. Spinal Cord Med.* 2004;27 Suppl 1:S88-92. PubMed PMID: 15503709.

[93] Mayfield JK, Erkkila JC, Winter RB. Spine deformity subsequent to acquired childhood spinal cord injury. *J. Bone Joint Surg. Am.* 1981;63(9):1401-11. PubMed PMID: 7320032.

In: Paraplegia
Editor: Agnes A. Holloway
ISBN: 978-1-63482-465-1

Chapter 3

ANAESTHETIC MANAGEMENT OF PATIENTS WITH CHRONIC SPINAL CORD INJURY

Alejandro Suarez-de-la-Rica** *and Iván Huercio
Department of Anaesthesiology and Critical Care H.U. La Paz, Madrid, Spain

ABSTRACT

Increasing numbers of patients with spinal cord injury (SCI) present for surgery or intrapartum care. A higher survival of these patients has lead to an increased prevalence and an increment in patients presenting for elective surgery. Managing these patients supposes a challenge to the anaesthesiologist.

Selection of a proper anaesthesia technique must prevent essentially autonomic hyperreflexia (AH), which may occur mainly with complete lesions above T7 (incidence of 85% in those patients), as it is more frequent in patients with higher lesions. Likelihood of triggering AH is essential to choose an anaesthetic technique. This condition consists on massive autonomic response caused by stimuli below the level of the injury, mainly pelvic visceral stimulation. Up to 82% of AH episodes are caused by bladder distension. Cutaneous and proprioceptive stimuli are less commonly responsible for this phenomenon. Surgery is a potent stimulus that could also provoque this condition, mostly in patients with

* Email of corresponding author: alejandro.suarez.delarica@gmail.com

previous history of AH or cervical lesions. Urological surgery is the most frequent procedure causing it.

Patients with frequent spasms normally require anaesthesia to undergo surgery as they are frequently triggered by proprioceptive and cutaneous stimuli, including surgical stimulus.

Many patients with low and complete lesions could undergo surgery without anaesthesia under the level of the lesion if AH is unlikely to occur and they are no troubled by daily spasms.

If anaesthesia is indicated, both general and regional anaesthesia could be used. Due to a reduction in lean tissue mass because of muscular atrophy the volume of distribution for intravenous agents is diminished. Succinilcholine, as depolirising neuromuscular blocking agent, should not be used in the early phase of SCI with the exception of the first 72h.

Regional anaesthesia, mainly spinal anaesthesia, prevents AH and spasms but it may be difficult to assess the level of the block and to perform the technique due to previous spinal surgery or bone deformities. Spinal anaesthesia normally provides haemodynamic stability. Epidural anaesthesia may also be achieved, but it is less predictable as the epidural space is normally distorted in these patients.

AH is also a severe complication during pregnancy, labour and delivery. Epidural anaesthesia impedes the occurrence of AH with variable success. If the risk of AH is high, an epidural catheter may be placed before labour, and maintained up to 5 days after delivery, when the risk of developing AH has diminished.

Introduction

Increasing numbers of patients with spinal cord injury (SCI) present for surgery or intrapartum care. Improvement in the care of these patients in both acute and chronic phase has contributed to a higher survival and quality of life. The higher prevalence leads to frequent presentation for surgery due to their condition or intercurrent medical problems. Managing these patients in the perioperative period supposes a challenge to the anaesthesiologist.

Epidemiology

In industrialized countries, annual incidence of SCI is about 30 to 50 cases per million people and the prevalence of spinal cord injured people from 500 to 900 cases per million people [1-2]. The main reported causes for SCI are road traffic accidents, falls and sports.

PATHOPHYSIOLOGY

Autonomic Hyperreflexia (AH)

This condition consists on massive autonomic response caused by stimuli below the level of the injury, mainly pelvic visceral stimulation. It was described by Kurnick in 1956 [3, 4] Hypertension is the most common symptom but headache, sweating, cutaneous flushing above the level of the lesion and reflex bradycardia are very common [4-5]. Pallor and cutaneous coldness are seen under the level of the lesion due to sympathetic stimulation [6]. Nausea and Horner´s syndrome are less commonly seen. Severe complications, even fatal, have been reported owing to hypertensive crises: intracranial bleeding, seizures, coma, myocardial ischemia and cardiac failure [7-10]. Incidence is about 85% of those patients with a lesion higher than T7 [4, 11-12]. The beginning of symptoms could develop at any time from 3 weeks to 12 years after SCI [5,13-14].

Both loss of descending inhibition and modifications in connections inside the distal spinal cord are the responsible physiological mechanisms that explain this condition [3, 15-17]. The terminal boutons of fibers separated by spinal cord transection multiply inappropriately, what leads to not suitable sympathetic response without descending inhibition.

Plasma noradrenaline levels remain low during and after the acute phase after SCI, probably because of the reduction in sympathetic activity. Plasma noradrenaline and urinary noradrenaline metabolites levels increase in case of AH [4] but they do not reache those observed in non spinal cord injured patients [18]. Maybe these patients are more sensitive to the effects of noradrenaline.

75-82% of AH episodes are caused by bladder distension [5, 13]. Therapeutic interventions as intramuscular injections or bronchial aspiration could trigger this condition too [19-23]. Cutaneous stimuli are less commonly responsible for this phenomenon [4].

Withdrawal of the precipitating stimulus and upright position assumption may be enough to return blood pressure to baseline levels [4]. Nevertheless antihypertensive agents of rapid onset and short duration are necessary in many cases. Sublingual nifedipine, glyceryl trinitrate and α-adrenergic blocking agents as phentolamine have been recommended. Hydralazine is frequently used too. The α-adrenergic blocking agent prazosin and guanethidine are effective in prevention [24-25], as well as sublingual nifedipine before cystoscopy [26].

Other Cardiovascular Alterations

Cardiac output adaptation to exercise, stress and pain disappear [21, 27-31].

Orthostatic hypotension is quite frequent [30, 32]. Upright position causes an important decrease in cerebral blood flow. Due to a decreased renal perfusion, renin-angiotensin system is stimulated what contributes to hydrosaline retention [33].

Persistence of non- counterbalanced parasympathetic activity may produce bradycardia episodes, even asystolia, during reflexogenic activities [20, 34-35]. Blood pressure baseline levels are lower than those of healthy people [18].

Respiratory Changes

Respiratory complications increase morbidity and mortality in spinal cord-injured patients because of bronchopulmonary infections and atelectasis. In case of T7-T10 injury, abdominal wall muscles paralysis severely impairs the ability to cough [36]. In T1-T7 lesions, due to impairment of accessory inspiratory muscles a restrictive syndrome is produced [37-40]. Cervical inspiratory muscles typically become hypertrophic and cervical perimeter is increased [41].

Gastrointestinal Changes

In patients with high lesions, gastric emptying is delayed, even in the chronic phase [42].

Urinary Complications

They are the second cause of mortality in spinal cord- injured patients [43]. In the chronic phase, mainly in incomplete lesions, reflex vesical activity may occur, without descendent coordination control, what may lead to vesical-sphincter dissinergy. This condition could provoke vesicoureteral reflux and urinary infections [43].

Allergic Risk

In spinal cord-injured patients there is no more latex sensibilitation in spite of a more frequent exposition [44].

Temperature

In high spinal lesions, mechanisms of thermoregulation are impaired because of the interruption of neuronal pathways to and from the hypothalamus. Body temperature depends on environmental one [45].

Although injury to these pathways should impair patient´s ability to mount a febrile response, in clinical practice fever is produced during infection in spinal cord-injured patients [46].

Muscle Disorders

Depolarising muscle relaxants usage following SCI may produce fatal increases in serum potassium concentrations. This was first published in 1970, with the description of four cases of cardiac arrest in paraplegic patients after the administration of succinylcholine [47]. The peak increase in potassium concentrations occurs 14 days after SCI [48]. Precurarisation with non-depolarising muscle relaxants may reduce potassium concentration increase [49].

Spasticity develops below the level of the lesion after the spinal shock phase, normally three or four months after injury. Spasms may be triggered by any minor stimulus and can be very violent. As spasticity prevents osteoporosis and increases venous return, treatment is only indicated if interference with daily life is present. The GABA agonist baclofen is useful in this kind of patients. Spasticity could develop kyphoscoliosis and other deformities.

Cutaneous Alterations

Pressure sores are frequent complications that occur in up to 60% of patients with cervical SCI due to immobility and anesthesia. Patiens suffering them frequently undergo surgery for debridement and closure [50]. They may trigger spasms or even AH.

Other Alterations

The risk of deep vein thrombosis is very high in the acute phase so prophylaxis is imperative.

Up to 52.3% of patients suffer anaemia, normally normochromic and normocytic due to chronic conditions [51].

Osteoporosis occurs throughout the body, specially in the pelvis. After 16 months of SCI, the reduction in bone density is maximum [52].

Chronic Pain

65-80% of patients develop chronic pain in the chronic phase of SCI and is normally difficult to manage it [53-55].

Anaesthetic Management

Orthopedic interventions, pressures sores debridement and closure and urologic surgery (lithiasis, urinary derivations) are the most frequent surgeries. In patients with complete lesions, with low likelihood of AH (lumbar lesions, without history of previous AH) and no frequent spasms scheduled for surgery under the level of the injury, sedation and local anesthesia administration may be an option.

Patients with frequent spasms normally require anaesthesia to undergo surgery as they are frequently triggered by proprioceptive and cutaneous stimuli, including surgical stimulus.

General Anaesthesia

Premedication

Premedication should be prescribed carefully, as patients with higher lesions may be sensitive to standard doses [56].

Haemodynamic Management

Vascular filling need to be adaptated in each patient since a reduced blood volume and an alteration in adaptative mechanisms to hypo and hypervolemia are present in these kind of patients. They are unable to compensate blood loss. Vasopressors may be used, but reactivity to them is unpredictable. Several studies suggest enhanced alpha-adrenoceptor responsiveness [34, 57]. Invasive blood pressure monitoring may be employed in the case of high hemorrhagic risk surgery but it is not necessary on a routine basis.

Airway Management

In spite of delayed gastric emptying, asymptomatic patients are not considered full stomach patients if preoperative fasting is respected. If severe gastroparesis is present, a rapid sequence induction is necessary. Erythromycin has been proposed as prokinetic agent to accelerate gastric emptying [58]. Orotracheal intubation may be difficult in cervical lesions and could provoke bradycardia, what can be prevented with administration of atropine [11, 59]. Hambly et al. reported a frequent laryngeal mask airway usage as alternative to tracheal tube in patients who underwent general anesthesia [60].

Intraoperative Pharmacology

Different studies found pharmacokinetic modifications in spinal cord-injured patients. Distribution volume is increased for aminoglycosides, and biodisponibility is decreased for theophyline and lorazepam [61-63].

There is almost no evidence related to anesthethic agents. Sevoflurane requirement is reduced by 20-39% during surgery below the level of the injury, probably due to a reduction in painful sensation. Sympathoadrenal response is reduced during and after surgery too [64]. So dose of any anesthethic agent must be titrated and adapted according to clinical response and bispectral index monitoring. Target controlled infusion (TCI) has no validated pharmacokinetic models in these patients, therefore it should not be used. The reduced blood volume and lean tissue mass implies a smaller volume of distribution for intravenous agents and a higher sensitivity to them [56]. They are not able to compensate for myocardial depressant effects neither. In a survey published bt Hambly et al. [60] propofol was the preferred induction agent. Presence of chronic renal failure may affect drug clearance too.

Analgesia should be effective enough to prevent AH during all the perioperative period. Muscle relaxant may not be necessary for surgery in case of important amiotrophy, but if orotracheal intubation is performed, muscle relaxation is normally employed. Curarization monitoring is recommended when employed [65]. Excitability changes are produced in motor axons under the level of the injury [66], then neuromuscular monitoring must be employed over the level of the lesion. In paraplegic patients, usual adductor pollicis monitoring may be used, but in tetraplegic patients orbicularis oculli monitoring is normally used.

During the period of denervation injury depolarizing muscle relaxants could induce severe hyperkalemia and even cardiac arrest [49, 67-69]. Succinylcholine is contraindicated in this period. In the first 72 h after the injury it may be safe [48-49]. It may be safely used again after 6 months [49], 9 months [15] or after 18 months [11] according to different authors. Rocuronium, a non-depolarizing neuromuscular blocker introduced in 1996, is capable of immediately establishing good intubating conditions as succinylcholine. So in rapid sequence induction rocuronium is a good alternative, but its employement contains a risk if the patient cannot be ventilated or oxygenated, that may be decreased with the recent introduction in 2008 of sugammadex for rapid reversal of rocuronium. Several studies have shown that rocuronium-sugammadex combination is faster than succinylcholine regarding recovery time of spontaneous ventilation [70-72] in case of impossibility to intubate the patient.

Intraoperative AH Management

Urological surgery is the most frequent procedure causing it [60]. If AH occurs during the perioperative period, removal of the precipitating stimulus may be enough. If AH persists, assuming the upright position and anesthesia deepening will allow to control AH in most cases [20, 35]. Antihypertensive agents must be used in refractory cases. As hypertensive crisis is normally quite short agents of rapid onset and short duration are preferred. Calcium channel blockers are frequently used for this indication. α-adrenergic blocking agents, nitrates, clonidine and urapidil have been successfully employed [5, 20, 35]. Per os or sublingual captopril may be useful too [73-74].

Positioning and Prevention of Hypothermia

Positioning must be carefully achieved. Padding at all pressure points is crucial. A gelatin cover is recommended.

Spinal cord patients are very prone to develop hypothermia, so prevention with fluid warming and hot air blankets is advised.

Spasms

Spasms in case of light anesthesia may occur due to surgical stimuli and anesthesia deepening is usually enough to control them. In one series spasms occurred in 6.9% of patients [60].

Mechanical Ventilation

Positive pressure ventilation may induce hypotension, mostly in case of higher lesions and in combination with myocardial depressant drugs [32]. Spontaneous ventilation is suitable for short procedures.

Locoregional Anaesthesia

Both spinal and epidural anesthesia are effective in preventing AH [11, 75] and spasms. Performing neuroaxial anesthesia could be technically complicated due to spinal anatomical distortion, previous surgery and inability to flex the spine because of spasms and deformities [76]. In lesions above T5, difficulties are less commonly found. In Schonwald et al. series, spinal anesthesia could be achieved in all patients with lesions above T5 [77]. Performing the puncture in lateral decubitus is preferable due to an easier positioning of the patient. Neurological outcome is not affected by neuroaxial blockade [11, 77].

Determining the level of the block may be very difficult. Observing where spasticity disappears may be very useful [78].

The low basal sympathetic tone is probably responsible for the cardiovascular stability normally obtained with spinal anesthesia in these patients [75, 79].

More failures are reported after epidural anesthesia, although it is theoretically as effective as spinal anesthesia for preventing AH [77, 79-80]. Distortion of epidural space and consequent non-uniform distribution, and the difficulty of assessing a test dose are possible explanations of these failures [77]. Adrenaline usage for test dose is not recommended as it could trigger AH.

Brachial plexus block is a useful anesthetic technique for upper limb surgery. In patients with cervical lesions, the nerve stimulator technique may be difficult to achieve if roots of brachial plexus have been damaged.

Analgesia and Anaesthesia in Obstetrics

The high incidence of SCI that affect women makes it an important issue to take into account for the obstetric and anesthetic management. It is even more important since more than 50% of the new cases occur for people between 16 and 30 years old, with women being 18% of this range [81].

The integration of these patients in social activities and improved programmes of rehabilitation, as it is for modern assisted reproductive techniques, may increase the number of women with chronic spinal cord injury that could consider pregnancy. Anesthesiologists should manage these patients focusing carefully on the particular aspects of the pathophysiology and the peri-operative concerns.

The medical conditions for women who present SCIs that may be aggravated by the physiological changes during pregnancy include cardiovascular, respiratory, hematologic, urogenital and dermatologic complications [82].

The level of the lesion has also to be considered prior to any anaesthetic procedure. Women with spinal cord transection below the T10 segment may have pain during labor. Those who have the lesion below S2 are likely to have bladder, bowel and sexual dysfunction. Patients with lesions above T10 are not likely to feel any labor pain, although those women with incomplete lesions between T5-T10 may feel pain if the spinal tracts are not damaged. Lesions above T5-T6 increase the risk of respiratory disorders and autonomic hyperreflexia. Depending on the level of the lesion and the progression of labor the anesthetic technique should be individually considered for each patient and obstetric context [83].

Medical Complications Aggravated by Pregnancy

Respiratory Changes

The reduction of expiratory reserve volume and functional residual capacity in the ventilatory parameters that physiologically occur during pregnancy, plus the increased need for minute ventilation, can aggravate the respiratory insufficiency that is associated with SCI. Decreased respiratory reserve and abdominal and intercostal muscle weakness caused by the cord injury, can impair the ability to cough, leading to atelectasis and respiratory infections [60, 83-85].

Cardiovascular Complications

Autonomic hyperreflexia (AH): Patients with chronic spinal cord injury experience autonomic hyperreflexia in 85% of the cases with injuries above T7. Approximately, 85-90% of the parturients with lesion above T6 are at risk of AH during labor [84]. It is not likely between T5-T8 and it is uncommon below T8. The noxius stimuli transmitted through the afferent nerves to the dorsal horn of the cord below the lesion, usually as a bladder, urethra or bowel distension or uterine contraction, can synapse with the sympathetic connections of the cord and paraspinal sympathetic chain. The consequent activation causes hyperactivity of the sympathetic system that is transmitted both craneally and caudally originating a situation of vasoconstriction that causes severe systemic hypertension and visceral spasm. The vasoconstriction at the area of the uterus can cause bradycardia and fetal hypoxia. Regarding the pregnant women, complications due to this great increase in blood pressure may lead to arrythmias (AV blocks and sinus arrest), intracraneal hemorrhage, hypertensive encephalopathy, and myocardial infarction. Not only labor and delivery can trigger the episode of AH, but also vaginal instrumentation, amniotomy, oxytocin infusion and perineal muscles distention should be considered as predisposing conditions [86-87].

Hypotension: The decreased systemic vascular resistance that pregnant women normally present, may be not satisfactorily compensated when orthostatic changes in blood pressure occur in cord injured patients. Those patients could have lost the ability to maintain the auto-regulation of the autonomous system as the cardiac sympathetic fibers (T1-T4) and splanchnic vasoconstriction efferent nerves (T5-L1) may be altered. This can impair the adequate utero-placental perfusion.

Hematological Changes

Anemia: Normochromic and normocytic anemia is not an uncommon condition in cord injured patients, and can be aggravated by the decreased hematocrit that appears during normal pregnancy.

Thromboembolism and deep vein thrombosis: The risk in cord injured patients is increased, particularly in the first stages, and can be developed in 80-85% of untreated patients.

Urogenital Complications

Chronic urinary tract infections: In cord injured patients, dyssynergy between the vesical muscles can create a lack of total urine voiding with vesicoureteral reflux that may lead to infections in the urinary tract. With regard to pregnant women, the physiological and hormonal changes can also increase the chance of urinary tract infections.

Urinary tract calculi and renal insufficiency: The vesicoureteral reflux, can also be a factor for formation of calculi which may predispose to urinary infections, proteinuria and eventually renal failure.

Dermatologic Changes

Pressure sores are a common complication in cord injured patients. This condition may be aggravated by the increased body weight in pregnant women.

Obstetric Considerations

Pregnant women with lesions above T11 have a higher rate of preterm labor [82]. It is recommended to use a cardiotocographer to monitor any fetal suffering, and it is even more important if autonomic hyperreflexia is likely, since it can impair uteroplacental blood supply [81]. Women may give birth vaginally, and assisted delivery may be necessary during the second stage of labor due to the inability for women to push [82]. Weekly cervical examinations after the 28th week are recommended and admission to hospital and obstetric control if cervical dilation is presented. It is also important to avoid, to the extent possible, any stimuli or distention while manipulating the vagina, urethra or bowel in order to prevent AH.

Anaesthetic Management

AH is the most threatening condition that should be taken into consideration in pregnant women with spinal cord injury before any anaesthetic practice. Labor should be considered as a potent stimulus that can trigger an episode of AH, and it should also be contemplated as a risk factor even in cord injured women with no previous history of AH. Therefore, it is strongly recommended to continuously monitor all high risk patients. It can be differentiated from any other obstetric hypertensive condition, as symptoms of AH are concomitant to uterine contractions [88]. Thus, when monitored, blood pressure may increase as contractions occur, and it may drop consequently when contractions diminish.

An antepartum consultation to establish the anaesthetic procedure and choose the most optimal technique for labor and delivery is also essential.

Regional Blocks: Epidural and Spinal Techniques

Neuraxial techniques are the preferred anesthetic procedures to manage anaesthesia and analgesia in pregnant cord injured patients, even though it may be difficult to success with the block. Because of their aggravated conditions, avoiding orthostatic hypotension by positioning the patient in a lateral decubitus may be a recommendable option prior to the administration of the anaesthetic dose. Assessing the blockade can also be a difficult situation, since the loss of sensitivity can only be assessed if it reaches a higher level above the cord lesion. However, as previously stated, it has been proposed to estimate the level of the block by evaluating the spinal segmental reflexes, since they will be absent below the block when it is completely achieved [78]

Due to the fact that cord injured patients have a predisposing haemodynamic instability, it has also be suggested to continuously monitor blood pressure by inserting an intra-arterial canula for labor and delivery prior to induction of anesthesia.

There is no contraindication to perform neuraxial techniques in patients with spinal anatomical abnormalities (even with surgical corrected spines) in paraplegic patients, even though the incidence of failure, dural puncture and patchy blockade with the epidural technique may be higher. However, the deleterious effect of the epidural on respiratory functions may be less likely than with intrathecal anesthesia.

Epidural analgesia is the most common neuraxial technique used to prevent the AH in cord injured women in the intrapartum. It can also be used to control postpartum pain, and decrease the likelihood to AH initiated by any noxious stimulus after labor. It is a satisfactory choice of analgesia since autonomic dysrreflexia has been reported to appear within the first 5 days after delivery [89].

Different combinations of local anaesthetics and opioids have been successfully demonstrated to treat and prevent AH. Meperidine, which has local anesthetic properties [90], bupivacaine 0.25% or 0.5%, and bupivacaine 0.25% plus fentanyl or morphine, have been reported to be effective to treat and prevent AH, whereas the use of fentanyl alone failed to control the symptoms [91]. Administration of local anaesthetic should be done cautiously with top-up doses through the epidural catheter, since it is difficult to assess the level of the blockade in cord injured patients. Thus, test dose may also be ineffective to assess subarachnoid injection of local anaesthetic. A nerve stimulator connected to an epidural catheter to confirm the correct epidural placement has also been proposed as an affective alternative [92].

Spinal analgesia and anaesthesia is another suitable neuraxial technique for cord injured patients to avoid any symptoms of AH. The use of continuous analgesia by using a spinal catheter may be a more suitable option in order to titrate the effect and avoid any unexpected complications [60]. Combined spinal-epidural technique has also been proposed as a choice for paraplegic pregnant women [93-94]. Since intrathecal analgesia and anaesthesia has a quicker onset of action, it can be a more suitable option if an urgent cesarean section is indicated by the obstetrician. However if it is administered in a single dose, a hypotensive response is more likely to occur than with an epidural technique [95].

General Anaesthesia

General anesthesia is not as common as the neuraxial techniques for analgesia and anaesthesia for labor in women with spinal cord injury. The use of general anesthesia in these type of patients may be indicated if regional blockade is not possible or successful, or severe respiratory insufficiency is present, so an optimal support of patient's ventilation can be achieved [96]. The use of depolarizing muscle relaxants, such as succinylcholine, is another important issue to take into account before general anesthesia. Depolarazing muscle relaxants are not recommended during the period of denervation injury, because there is an increased risk of secondary severe hyperkalemia [97]. Nondepolarizing agents can safely be used instead for intubation since there is no contraindication for cord injured women.

Intravenous antihypertensive agents can also be used if regional techniques fail, in order to avoid the symptoms of AH, but they always have to be used carefully in order to avoid hypotension and a consequent decrease in utero-placental blood supply [98]. Arteriolar vasodilators, magnesium sulfate, beta-adrenergic blockers, sodium nitroprusside (precisely adjusting the dose for potential fetal cyanide intoxication), may be used for preventing or treating the symptomatic response to AH.

CONCLUSION

Spinal cord-injured patients have a higher survival and quality of life, what have determined that an increasing number of patients present for surgery or labor. In spite of their hypo or anesthesia below the level of the lesion, an adequate anesthetic technique must be chosen in order to avoid autonomic hyperreflexia and spasms. Both general and regional anaesthesia may contribute to a correct perioperative or intrapartum management.

REFERENCES

[1] Amar AP, Levy ML. Surgical controversies in the management of spinal cord injury. *J. Am. Coll Surg.,* 1999;188:550-66.

[2] McDonald JW, Sadowsky C. Spinal-cord injury. Lancet 2002;359:417-25.

[3] Kurnick NB. Autonomic hyperreflexia and its control in patients with spinal cord lesions. *Ann. Intern. Med.,* 1956;44:678-86.

[4] Colachis SC, 3rd. Autonomic hyperreflexia with spinal cord injury. *J. Am. Paraplegia Soc.,* 1992;15:171-86.

[5] Lindan R, Joiner E, Freehafer AA, Hazel C. Incidence and clinical features of autonomic dysreflexia in patients with spinal cord injury. *Paraplegia,* 1980;18:285-92.

[6] Naftchi NE, Richardson JS. Autonomic dysreflexia: pharmacological management of hypertensive crises in spinal cord injured patients. *J. Spinal. Cord Med.,* 1997;20:355-60.

[7] Karlsson AK. Autonomic dysreflexia. *Spinal Cord,* 1999;37:383-91.

[8] Eltorai I, Kim R, Vulpe M, Kasravi H, Ho W. Fatal cerebral hemorrhage due to autonomic dysreflexia in a tetraplegic patient: case report and review. *Paraplegia,* 1992;30:355-60.

[9] Karlsson AK. Autonomic dysfunction in spinal cord injury: clinical presentation of symptoms and signs. *Prog. Brain Res.,* 2006;152:1-8.

[10] Valles M, Benito J, Portell E, Vidal J. Cerebral hemorrhage due to autonomic dysreflexia in a spinal cord injury patient. *Spinal Cord,* 2005;43:738-40.

[11] Amzallag M. Autonomic hyperreflexia. *Int. Anesthesiol. Clin.,* 1993;31: 87-102.

[12] Wanner MB, Rageth CJ, Zach GA. Pregnancy and autonomic hyperreflexia in patients with spinal cord lesions. *Paraplegia,* 1987;25 :482-90.

[13] Kewalramani LS. Autonomic dysreflexia in traumatic myelopathy. *Am. J. Phys. Med.,* 1980;59:1-21.

[14] Bors E. The challenge of quadriplegia; some personal observations in a series of two hundred thirty-three cases. *Bull Los Angel Neuro Soc.,* 1956; 21:105-23.

[15] Fraser A, Edmonds-Seal J. Spinal cord injuries. A review of the problems facing the anaesthetist. *Anaesthesia,* 1982;37:1084-98.

[16] Krassioukov AV, Weaver LC. Reflex and morphological changes in spinal preganglionic neurons after cord injury in rats. *Clin. Exp. Hypertens,* 1995;17:361-73.

[17] Krassioukov AV, Weaver LC. Episodic hypertension due to autonomic dysreflexia in acute and chronic spinal cord-injured rats. *Am. J. Physiol.,* 1995;268:H2077-83.

[18] Mathias CJ, Christensen NJ, Corbett JL, Frankel HL, Spalding JM. Plasma catecholamines during paroxysmal neurogenic hypertension in quadriplegic man. *Circ. Res.,* 1976;39:204-8.

[19] Mathias CJ. Bradycardia and cardiac arrest during tracheal suction--mechanisms in tetraplegic patients. *Eur. J. Intensive Care Med.,* 1976;2: 147-56.

[20] Blackmer J. Rehabilitation medicine: 1. *Autonomic dysreflexia. CMAJ,* 2003;169:931-5.

[21] Teasell RW, Arnold JM, Krassioukov A, Delaney GA. Cardiovascular consequences of loss of supraspinal control of the sympathetic nervous system after spinal cord injury. *Arch. Phys. Med. Rehabil.,* 2000;81:506-16.

[22] Laird AS, Carrive P, Waite PM. Cardiovascular and temperature changes in spinal cord injured rats at rest and during autonomic dysreflexia. *J. Physiol.,* 2006;577:539-48.

[23] Selcuk B, Inanir M, Kurtaran A, Sulubulut N, Akyuz M. Autonomic dysreflexia after intramuscular injection in traumatic tetraplegia: a case report. *Am. J. Phys. Med. Rehabil.,* 2004;83:61-4.

[24] Brown BT, Carrion HM, Politano VA. Guanethidine sulfate in the prevention of autonomic hyperreflexia. *J. Urol.,* 1979;122:55-7.

[25] Krum H, Louis W, Brown D, Howes L. A study of the alpha-1 adrenoreceptor blocker prazosin in the prophylactic management of autonomic dysreflexia in high spinal cord injury patients. *Clinical autonomic research,* 1992;2:83-8.

[26] Dykstra DD, Sidi AA, Anderson LC. The effect of nifedipine on cystoscopy-induced autonomic hyperreflexia in patients with high spinal cord injuries. *J. Urol.,* 1987;138:1155-7.

[27] Coutts KD, Rhodes EC, McKenzie DC. Maximal exercise responses of tetraplegics and paraplegics. *J. Appl. Physiol. Respir. Environ Exerc. Physiol.,* 1983;55:479-82.

[28] Eriksson P, Lofstrom L, Ekblom B. Aerobic power during maximal exercise in untrained and well-trained persons with quadriplegia and paraplegia. *Scand. J. Rehabil. Med.,* 1988;20:141-7.

[29] Frankel HL, Michaelis LS, Golding DR, Beral V. The blood pressure in paraplegia. I. *Paraplegia,* 1972;10:193-200.

[30] Gonzalez F, Chang JY, Banovac K, Messina D, Martinez-Arizala A, Kelley RE. Autoregulation of cerebral blood flow in patients with orthostatic hypotension after spinal cord injury. *Paraplegia,* 1991; 29:1-7.

[31] Lehmann KG, Lane JG, Piepmeier JM, Batsford WP. Cardiovascular abnormalities accompanying acute spinal cord injury in humans: incidence, time course and severity. *J. Am. Coll Cardiol.,* 1987;10:46-52.

[32] Alderson J. Chronic care of spinal cord injury. In: Alderson J, Frost E, eds. Spinal cord injuries Anaesthetic and associated care. London: Butterworth; 1990:104-25.

[33] Mathias CJ, Frankel HL. Cardiovascular control in spinal man. *Annu. Rev. Physiol.,* 1988;50:577-92.

[34] Mathias CJ, Frankel HL, Christensen NJ, Spalding JM. Enhanced pressor response to noradrenaline in patients with cervical spinal cord transection. *Brain,* 1976;99:757-70.

[35] Bycroft J, Shergill IS, Chung EA, Arya N, Shah PJ. Autonomic dysreflexia: a medical emergency. *Postgrad. Med. J.,* 2005;81:232-5.

[36] Chen CF, Lien IN, Wu MC. Respiratory function in patients with spinal cord injuries: effects of posture. *Paraplegia,* 1990;28:81-6.

[37] Ledsome JR, Sharp JM. Pulmonary function in acute cervical cord injury. *Am. Rev. Respir. Dis.,* 1981;124:41-4.

[38] Anke A, Aksnes AK, Stanghelle JK, Hjeltnes N. Lung volumes in tetraplegic patients according to cervical spinal cord injury level. *Scand. J. Rehabil. Med.,* 1993;25:73-7.

[39] Baydur A, Adkins RH, Milic-Emili J. Lung mechanics in individuals with spinal cord injury: effects of injury level and posture. *J. Appl. Physiol., (*1985) 2001;90:405-11.

[40] Brown R, DiMarco AF, Hoit JD, Garshick E. Respiratory dysfunction and management in spinal cord injury. *Respir. Care,* 2006;51:853-68;discussion 69-70.

[41] Frisbie JH, Brown R. Waist and neck enlargement after quadriplegia. *J. Am. Paraplegia Soc.,* 1994;17:177-8.

[42] Segal JL, Milne N, Brunnemann SR. Gastric emptying is impaired in patients with spinal cord injury. *Am. J. Gastroenterol.,* 1995;90:466-70.
[43] Siroky MB. Pathogenesis of bacteriuria and infection in the spinal cord injured patient. *Am. J. Med.,* 2002;113 Suppl 1A:67S-79S.
[44] Mertes PM, Mouton C, Fremont S, et al. Latex hypersensitivity in spinal cord injured adult patients. *Anaesth Intensive Care,* 2001;29:393-9.
[45] Petrofsky JS. Thermoregulatory stress during rest and exercise in heat in patients with a spinal cord injury. *Eur. J. Appl. Physiol. Occup. Physiol.,* 1992;64:503-7.
[46] Schmidt KD, Chan CW. Thermoregulation and fever in normal persons and in those with spinal cord injuries. *Mayo Clin. Proc.,* 1992;67: 469-75.
[47] Tobey RE. Paraplegia, succinylcholine and cardiac arrest. *Anesthesiology,* 1970;32:359-64.
[48] John DA, Tobey RE, Homer LD, Rice CL. Onset of succinylcholine-induced hyperkalemia following denervation. *Anesthesiology,* 1976;45:294-9.
[49] Gronert GA, Theye RA. Pathophysiology of hyperkalemia induced by succinylcholine. *Anesthesiology,* 1975;43:89-99.
[50] Parsons K, Stawiski M. Dermatologic complications of spinal cord injury. *Annual meeting of ASCA,* 1983.
[51] Perkash A, Brown M. Anaemia in patients with traumatic spinal cord injury. *Paraplegia,* 1982;20:235-6.
[52] Garland DE, Stewart CA, Adkins RH, et al. Osteoporosis after spinal cord injury. *J. Orthop. Res.,* 1992;10:371-8.
[53] Finnerup NB, Johannesen IL, Sindrup SH, Bach FW, Jensen TS. Pain and dysesthesia in patients with spinal cord injury: A postal survey. *Spinal Cord,* 2001;39:256-62.
[54] Yezierski RP. Spinal cord injury: a model of central neuropathic pain. *Neurosignals,* 2005;14:182-93.
[55] Beric A. Spinal cord injury pain. *Eur. J. Pain,* 2003;7:335-8.
[56] Goy J. Spinal injuries. In: Arnold E, ed. Orthopaedic Anaesthesia. London; 1994:145-57.
[57] Arnold JM, Feng QP, Delaney GA, Teasell RW. Autonomic dysreflexia in tetraplegic patients: evidence for alpha-adrenoceptor hyper-responsiveness. *Clin. Auton. Res.,* 1995;5:267-70.
[58] Clanton LJ, Jr., Bender J. Refractory spinal cord injury induced gastroparesis: resolution with erythromycin lactobionate, a case report. *J. Spinal Cord Med.,* 1999;22:236-8.

[59] Frankel HL, Mathias CJ, Spalding JM. Mechanisms of reflex cardiac arrest in tetraplegic patients. *Lancet,* 1975;2:1183-5.
[60] Hambly PR, Martin B. Anaesthesia for chronic spinal cord lesions. *Anaesthesia,* 1998;53:273-89.
[61] Segal JL, Brunnemann SR, Eltorai IM, Vulpe M. Decreased systemic clearance of lorazepam in humans with spinal cord injury. *J. Clin. Pharmacol.,* 1991;31:651-6.
[62] Segal JL, Brunnemann SR, Gordon SK, Eltorai IM. The absolute bioavailability of oral theophylline in patients with spinal cord injury. *Pharmacotherapy,* 1986;6:26-9.
[63] Segal JL, Brunnemann SR, Gordon SK, Eltorai IM. Amikacin pharmacokinetics in patients with spinal cord injury. *Pharmacotherapy,* 1988;8:79-81.
[64] Yoo K, Hwang J, Jeong S, et al. Anesthetic requirements and stress hormone responses in spinal cord-injured patients undergoing surgery below the level of injury. *Anesth Analg.,* 2006;102:1223-8.
[65] SFAR. Consensus conference. Indications for curarisation in anesthesia. *Ann. Fr. Anesth. Reanim.,* 2000;19:344-472.
[66] Lin CS, Macefield VG, Elam M, Wallin BG, Engel S, Kiernan MC. Axonal changes in spinal cord injured patients distal to the site of injury. *Brain,* 2007;130:985-94.
[67] Gronert GA. Use of suxamethonium in cord patients--whether and when. *Anaesthesia,* 1998;53:1035-6.
[68] Matthews JM. Succinylcholine-induced hyperkalemia. *Anesthesiology,* 2006;105:430; author reply 1.
[69] Yentis SM. Suxamethonium and hyperkalaemia. *Anaesth Intensive Care,* 1990;18:92-101.
[70] McCahon R. Role of sugammadex in rapid sequence induction and intubation. *Br. J. Anaesth,* 2012;109:123; author reply -4.
[71] Lee C, Jahr JS, Candiotti KA, Warriner B, Zornow MH, Naguib M. Reversal of profound neuromuscular block by sugammadex administered three minutes after rocuronium: a comparison with spontaneous recovery from succinylcholine. *Anesthesiology,* 2009; 110:1020-5.
[72] Sorensen MK, Bretlau C, Gatke MR, Sorensen AM, Rasmussen LS. Rapid sequence induction and intubation with rocuronium-sugammadex compared with succinylcholine: a randomized trial. *Br. J. Anaesth,* 2012;108:682-9.

[73] Anton HA, Townson A. Drug therapy for autonomic dysreflexia. CMAJ 2004;170:1210; author reply
[74] Esmail Z, Shalansky KF, Sunderji R, Anton H, Chambers K, Fish W. Evaluation of captopril for the management of hypertension in autonomic dysreflexia: a pilot study. *Arch. Phys. Med. Rehabil.,* 2002; 83:604-8.
[75] Barker I, Alderson J, Lydon M, Franks CI. Cardiovascular effects of spinal subarachnoid anaesthesia. A study in patients with chronic spinal cord injuries. *Anaesthesia,* 1985;40:533-6.
[76] Rocco A, Vandam L. Problems in anesthesia for paraplegics. *Anesthesiology,* 1959;20:348-54.
[77] Schonwald G, Fish KJ, Perkash I. Cardiovascular complications during anesthesia in chronic spinal cord injured patients. *Anesthesiology,* 1981;55:550-8.
[78] Stirt JA, Marco A, Conklin KA. Obstetric anesthesia for a quadriplegic patient with autonomic hyperreflexia. *Anesthesiology,* 1979;51:560-2.
[79] Broecker BH, Hranowsky N, Hackler RH. Low spinal anesthesia for the prevention of autonomic dysreflexia in the spinal cord injury patient. *J. Urol.,* 1979;122:366.
[80] Owen MD, Stiles MM, Opper SE, McNitt JD, Fibuch EE. Autonomic hyperreflexia in a pregnant paraplegic patient. Case report. *Reg. Anesth.,* 1994;19:415-7.
[81] ACOG Committee Opinion: Number 275, September 2002. Obstetric management of patients with spinal cord injuries. Obstet *Gynecol.,* 2002;100:625-7.
[82] Pereira L. Obstetric management of the patient with spinal cord injury. *Obstet. Gynecol. Surv.,* 2003;58:678-87.
[83] Crosby E, St-Jean B, Reid D, Elliott RD. Obstetrical anaesthesia and analgesia in chronic spinal cord-injured women. *Can. J. Anaesth,* 1992; 39:487-94.
[84] Kang AH. Traumatic spinal cord injury. *Clin. Obstet. Gynecol.,* 2005; 48:67-72.
[85] Bader A. Spinal cord injury. Neurologic and neuromuscular disease. In: Chestnut D, ed. Obstetric anesthesia principles and practice. 5th ed. Philadelphia; 2014:1056-8.
[86] Boucher M SL, Mernard L, Sabbah R. Epidural and labor in paraplegics. *Can. J. Obstet. Gynecol.,* 1991;3:130-2.
[87] Abouleish E. Hypertension in a paraplegic parturient. *Anesthesiology,* 1980;53:348.

[88] Rossier AB, Ruffieux M, Ziegler WH. Pregnancy and labour in high traumatic spinal cord lesions. *Paraplegia,* 1969;7:210-6.
[89] Cross LL, Meythaler JM, Tuel SM, Cross AL. Pregnancy, labor and delivery post spinal cord injury. *Paraplegia,* 1992;30:890-902.
[90] Baraka A. Epidural meperidine for control of autonomic hyperreflexia in a paraplegic parturient. *Anesthesiology,* 1985;62:688-90.
[91] Abouleish EI, Hanley ES, Palmer SM. Can epidural fentanyl control autonomic hyperreflexia in a quadriplegic parturient? *Anesth Analg.,* 1989;68:523-6.
[92] Riazi S, Niazi AU, Tumber PS, Peng P. Confirmation of epidural catheter placement in a quadriplegic patient using a nerve stimulator. *Can. J. Anaesth,* 2010;57:276-7.
[93] Kobayashi A, Mizobe T, Tojo H, Hashimoto S. Autonomic hyperreflexia during labour. *Can. J. Anaesth.,* 1995;42:1134-6.
[94] Agostoni M, Giorgi E, Beccaria P, Zangrillo A, Valentini G. Combined spinal-epidural anaesthesia for Caesarean section in a paraplegic woman: difficulty in obtaining the expected level of block. *Eur. J. Anaesthesiol.,* 2000;17:329-31.
[95] Ng K, Parsons J, Cyna AM, Middleton P. Spinal versus epidural anaesthesia for caesarean section. Cochrane *Database Syst. Rev.,* 2004:CD003765.
[96] Ahmed AB, Bogod DG. Anaesthetic management of a quadriplegic patient with severe respiratory insufficiency undergoing caesarean section. *Anaesthesia,* 1996;51:1043-5.
[97] Stone WA, Beach TP, Hamelberg W. Succinylcholine-induced hyperkalemia in dogs with transected sciatic nerves or spinal cords. *Anesthesiology,* 1970;32:515-20.
[98] Westgren N, Hultling C, Levi R, Westgren M. Pregnancy and delivery in women with a traumatic spinal cord injury in Sweden, 1980-1991. *Obstet Gynecol.,* 1993;81:926-30.

In: Paraplegia
Editor: Agnes A. Holloway

ISBN: 978-1-63482-465-1

Chapter 4

MORPHOLOGICAL CHANGES OF TOENAILS IN HEMIPLEGIA: TOENAIL CONFIGURATION IS DETERMINED BY THE MECHANICAL FORCES ON THE FOOT

Hitomi Sano* and Rei Ogawa
Department of Plastic, Reconstructive and Aesthetic Surgery, Nippon Medical School, Tokyo, Japan

ABSTRACT

Nails have numerous functions. Fingernails are important for protecting the distal phalanges, enhancing tactile discrimination, and performing fine manipulation. They are also used for scratching and grooming. Toenails protect the distal toes and contribute to pedal biomechanics. Thus, nails are frequently exposed on a daily basis to physical stimuli such as counter pressure and shear force. Our recent studies revealed that mechanical forces may have a particularly pronounced effect on nail configuration, and thus may be involved in the development of nail deformities. One such deformity is pincer nail, which is defined as the transverse overcurvature of the nail plate that increases

---

* Corresponding author's email: sasasa116sasasa@hotmail.com.

along the longitudinal axis. The known causative factors of pincer nail include heredity, inappropriate nail cutting, and, most commonly, poorly fitting shoes that impose inappropriate physical forces on the nail. However, our extensive clinical experience shows that patients with hemiplegia also frequently develop pincer nail on the palsied side, which receives weaker mechanical forces on a daily basis than the non-palsied side. At present, however, this phenomenon is poorly documented and understood.

This chapter reviews the effect of mechanical force on nail configuration and introduces our studies on the morphological changes of the toenails in patients with hemiplegia.

When the curvature of the great toenails on the palsied and non-palsied sides of subjects with hemiplegia was measured, the great toenail on the palsied side was found to be significantly more curved than the great toenail on the non-palsied side. This phenomenon was also observed in the mouse model of hemiplegia, which was generated by cutting the sciatic nerve in the left hin dleg of each mouse to create a denervated leg. One month after the operation, the denervated and innervated hind legs were evaluated macroscopically and histologically. The third toenails of the denervated legs were significantly more curved in the short and long axis than the third toenails of the innervated legs.

Understanding the relationship between mechanical force and nail configuration could revolutionize the treatment of nail deformities. This relationship suggests that nail deformities could be prevented and treated by eliminating excessive mechanical forces, by increasing mechanical forces, or by limiting the inherent tendency of the nail to curve, which counteracts daily downward mechanical forces. An example of the latter approach is softening the nail by applying an external preparation or thinning the nail with a nail rasp. We hope that the information contained in this review will help to inform and initiate future experimentation on the roles that mechanical forces play in the functions of our bodies, including our nails.

1. Introduction

Mechanical stimuli play an important role in cell proliferation and differentiation, and in tissue degeneration and development. The study of the biological effects of these mechanical stimuli is called mechanobiology, which is a rapidly emerging field [1-5]. Classic examples of the mechanical stimuli that are placed on cells and tissues are those that occur during walking. When a human being walks, the feet are subjected to various mechanical forces, including counter pressure from the plantar and/or shear force from the shoes.

Walking is divided into two phases, namely, the stance and swing phases. The stance phase consists of "heel strike" followed by "foot flat", "mid-stance", "heel off", and finally "toe off". The swing phase is a continuous phase that starts from "toe off", shifts to "mid-swing", and ends with "heel strike", which finishes the walking cycle. Walking consists of repeats of this cycle [6]. Each of the components of these walking phases associates with a specific type, force, and angle of mechanical stimulation of the tissues of the foot.

When patients with hemiplegia seek to walk, they must compensate for the palsy on one side by adopting certain gaits. A typical gait pattern of patients with hemiplegic cerebral palsy is toe-walking, which is defined as walking on the toes of the affected side without putting much weight on the heel or any other part of the foot [7-10]. However, such compensatory gait changes can cause secondary problems and alter the gait pattern further.

2. Role of Mechanical Force in Nail Configuration

Toenails are important for protecting the distal toes and contributing to pedal biomechanics. In normal circumstances, they are exposed on a daily basis to mechanical stimuli such as counter pressure and shear force. Recent studies show that such mechanical forces particularly affect nail configuration and that when they are inadequate or excessive, they can promote the development of nail deformities [11-15]. Specifically, when the nails of toes or fingers receive less physical stimulation than normal, they tend to curve inward. Conversely, the nails of toes and fingers that undergo a lot of physical stimulation tend to have a flat or concave shape. For example, the degree of toenail curvature in bedridden patients tends to increase as the duration of the bedridden state rises; this effect is the result of lack of mechanical force on the toenail [13]. Conversely, the nails of toes and fingers that undergo a lot of physical stimulation tend to have a flat or concave shape. For example, excessive mechanical force on the toe or finger pads is responsible for koilonychias, which is characterized by spooning of the nails [14-15].

Pincer nail is a commonly observed nail deformation and is defined as the transverse over curvature of the nail plate that increases along the longitudinal axis. The classical causative factors of pincer nail include heredity, inappropriate physical forces due to ill-fitting shoes, and inappropriate nail cutting. However, our studies show that pincer nail can also be caused by the lack of upward mechanical forces on the finger or toe pad.

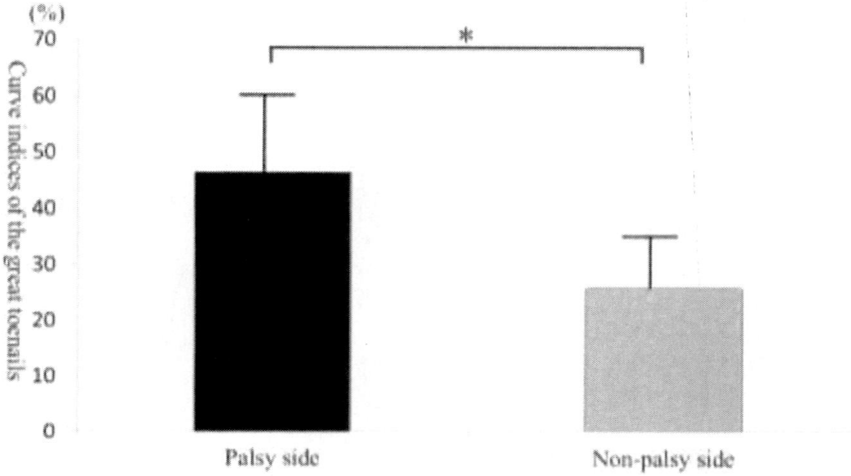

*p < 0.01.

Figure 1. Mean curve indices of the great toenails on the palsied and non-palsied sides of hemiplegia cases. On average, the great toenail on the palsied side had a significantly higher curve index than the great toenail on the non-palsied side.

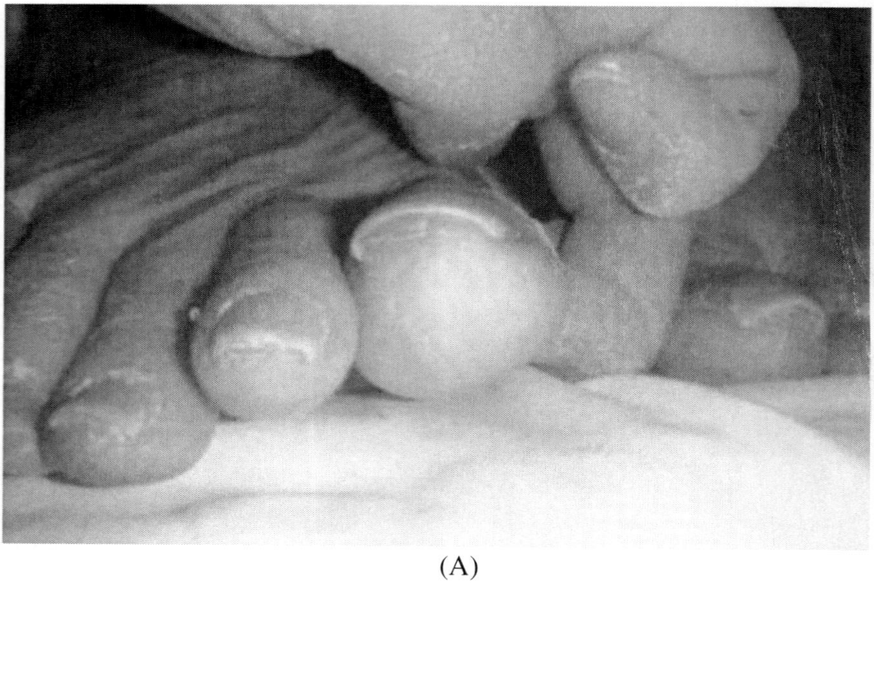

(A)

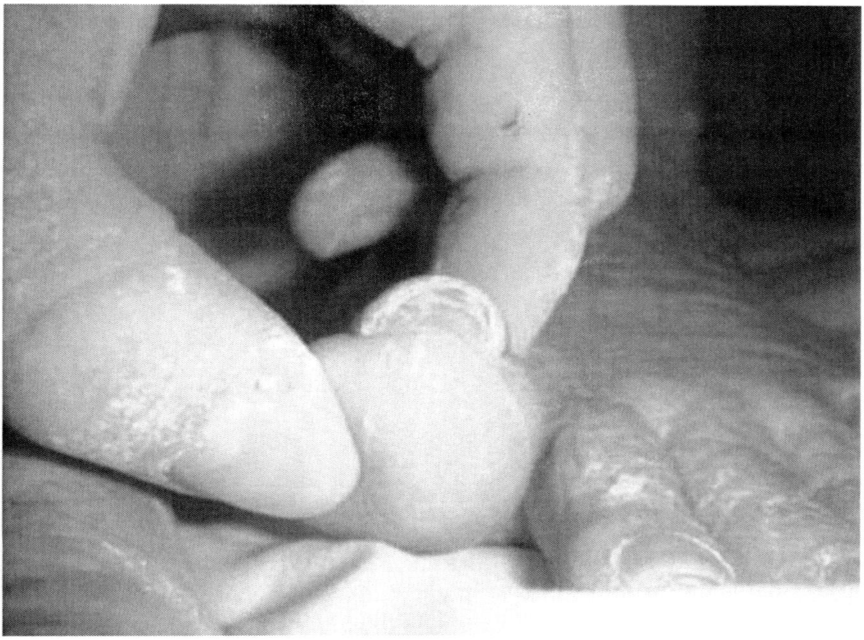

(B)

Figure 2. Typical findings in hemiplegia. The great toenails of an 83-year-old female with hemiplegia after cerebral infarction that had occurred 4 years earlier are shown. The great toenail on the palsied side shows greater inward curvature than the great toenail on the non-palsied side.

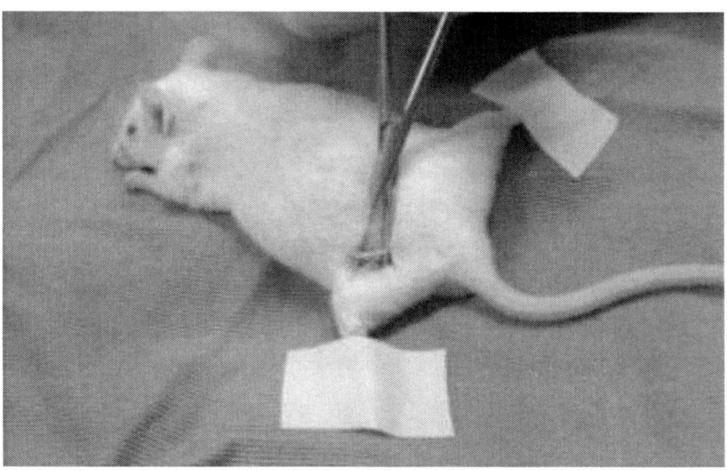

Figure 3. Animal model of hemiplegia. The sciatic nerve in the left hind leg was cut and a 10 mm piece was excised.

3. Our Recent Studies

The palsied side of patients with complete hemiplegia (Brunnstrom motor deficit stage I) is subjected to relatively weaker mechanical forces than the non-palsied side. This led us to hypothesize that this disparity between the palsied and non-palsied side would lead to morphological changes in the toenails. To test this, we performed two studies. The clinical study involved measuring the curvature of the great toenails of the palsied and non-palsied sides of subjects with hemiplegia. The experimental study involved an animal model of hemiplegia, in which one leg was denervated. One month after the operation, the third toenail curvature of the denervated and innervated legs was measured.

3.1. Clinical Study of Patients with Hemiplegia

The study sample consisted of the 20 great toenails of ten subjects (two males, eight females; mean age 82 ± 6.0 years). All had had hemiplegia for more than 3 months (the average duration of hemiplegia was 25.5 ± 11.4 months) due to cerebrovascular disease. All had Brunnstrom motor deficit stage I hemiplegia. All participants were provided with a thorough explanation about the purpose and method of this study, and all gave their consent to participate. The procedures were consistent with the revised Helsinki Declaration of 1983. Subjects with factors that have been reported to affect nail morphology [16] were excluded. These factors were treatment with β-blockers, corticosteroids or immunosuppressive agents, radiation therapy, or chemotherapy, and the presence of anemia, psoriasis, tinea infection, subungual hematoma, or traumatic or congenital deformity.

The palsied and non-palsied sides were compared in terms of great toenail morphology. The nail configuration was assessed by determining the curve index (defined as [nail height/nail width] *100 (%)) and the nail thickness. The curve index was calculated by using digital photo images of the front of the great toes. All data were summarized as means ± SD. The two groups were compared in terms of curve index or nail thickness by paired Student's t-test. $P < 0.05$ was considered to indicate statistical significance. The great toenail on the palsied side had a higher curve index than the great toenail on the non-palsied side in all cases. This difference was statistically significant (46.5 ± 14.6% *vs.* 25.9 ± 10.0%, $p < 0.01$) (Figure 1). Figure 2 shows typical findings in a case with hemiplegia. This patient was an 83-year-old female with hemiplegia after a cerebral infarction that had occurred 4 years earlier. The great toenail on the palsied side (A, curve index = 58.0%) showed greater inward curvature than the great toenail on the non-palsied side (B, curve index = 30.4%).

3.2. Experimental Study with a Hemiplegia Mouse Model

Six 7-week-old ICR mice (Crea Japan Inc, Tokyo, Japan) were anesthetized, and the sciatic nerve of the left hind leg of each mouse was cut, and a 10 mm piece was excised (Figure 3). The right leg remained innervated and served as a control. Thirty days after the operation, the animals were sacrificed, and the denervated and innervated hind legs were evaluated macroscopically and histologically. The nail curvature on the long axis was calculated by using digital photo images of the side of the third toes. The nail curvature on the long axis was assessed by determining the angle between the tangents of the nail curve and the curve of the hyponychium, which is the epidermal ridge that demarcates the junction between the finger pulp and the subungual structures. The third toenails on both sides were harvested together with part of the first joint of each toe. Each tissue specimen was fixed with zinc-fixative solution (IHC Zinc Fixative, BD Pharmingen, Tokyo, Japan) and embedded in paraffin. Hematoxylin and eosin (H & E) staining was used to detect the curve on the short axis. The curve on the short axis was defined as the angle between the tangents of both sides of the curve that started the vertex. The denervated and innervated legs were compared in terms of third toenail curvature in the long or short axis by paired Student's t-test. $P < 0.05$ was considered to indicate statistical significance. The denervated legs had significantly more curved third toenails in the long ($71.1 \pm 5.7°$ *vs.* $112.7 \pm 10.6°$) (Figure 4) and short axes ($73.3 \pm 14.4°$ *vs.* $108.5 \pm 9.5°$) than the innervated legs (Figure 5). Typical macroscopic and microscopic findings of the third toenails of the hemiplegia model mice are shown in Figures 6 and 7.

4. Discussion and Future Perspectives

Hemiplegia cases have a high incidence of unilateral pincer nail. This can be explained by the relationship between mechanical force and nail configuration: the reduction of mechanical force on the toe pads of the palsied side means that the inherent tendency of nails to curve upward is no longer counterbalanced, leading to excessive toenail curvature on the palsied side. This notion is supported by our clinical study: the great toenail of the palsied side curved significantly more strongly than the great toenail of the non-palsied sides. Moreover, the hemiplegia animal model study showed that compared to the toenails on the innervated leg, the third toenail of the denervated leg curved more strongly inward in both the short and long axes 1 month after denervation.

The over-curved nails of patients with hemiplegia can become clinically problematic. In particular, their shape could lead to inappropriate (e.g., too short) nail cutting, which could easily lead to inflammation. To prevent such nail trouble, medical personnel and caregivers should be aware of the causes of nail deformities and implement appropriate nail care methods.

The mechanobiology theory described above could also revolutionize the prevention and treatment of nail deformities. For example, it may be possible to prevent or treat nail deformity by applying mechanical force externally in the form of massage, or shape-memory wire. Alternative approaches to preventing or treating nail deformities are to counteract the inherent tendency of nails to curve upward by softening the nail with external medication or by thinning the nails with a rasp.

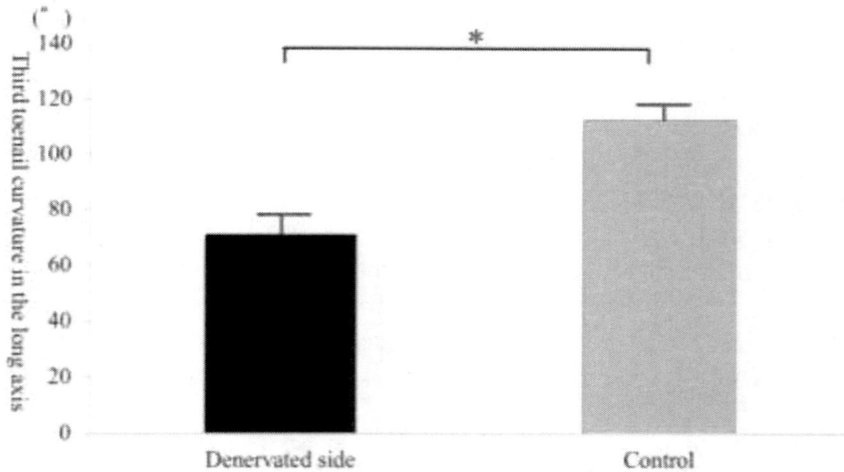

*p < 0.01.

Figure 4. Mean third toenail curvature in the long axis of hemiplegia model mice. On average, 1 month after left sciatic nerve denervation, the third toenail of the denervated leg was significantly more curved in the long axis than the third toenail of the innervated leg.

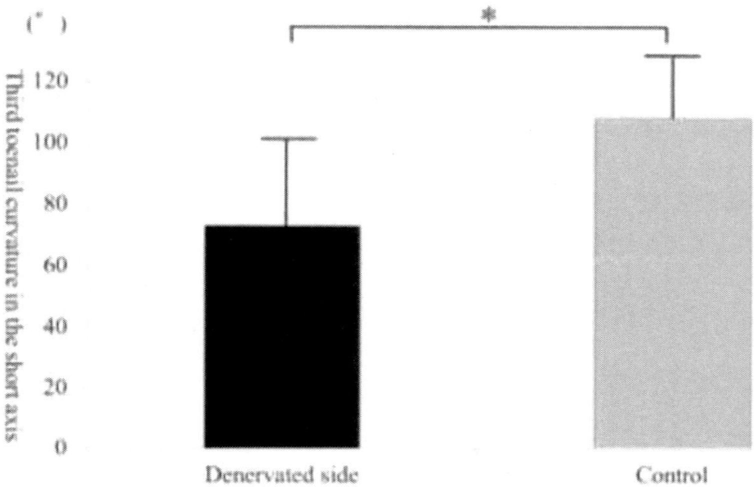

Figure 5. Mean third toenail curvature in the short axis of hemiplegia model mice. On average, 1 month after left sciatic nerve denervation, the third toenail of the denervated leg was significantly more curved in the short axis than the third toenail of the innervated leg.

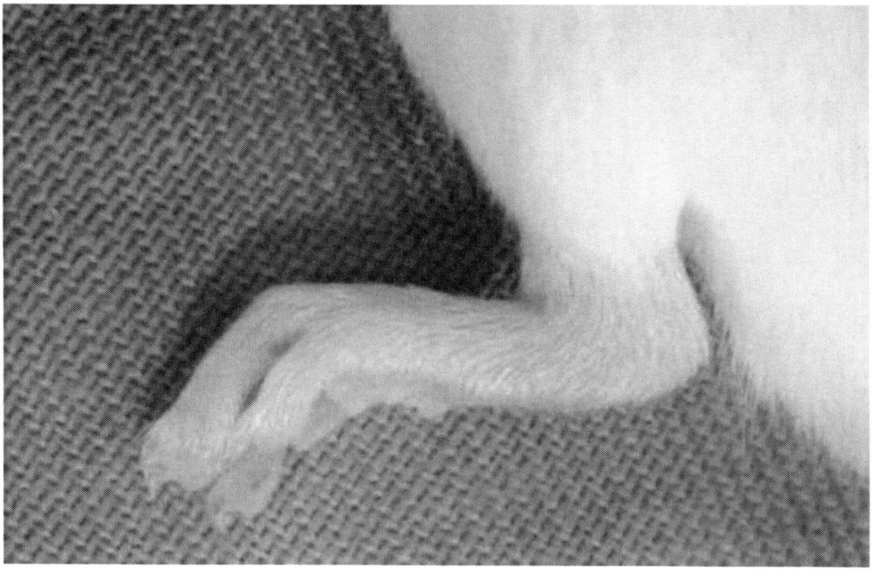

(A)

Figure 6. (Continued)

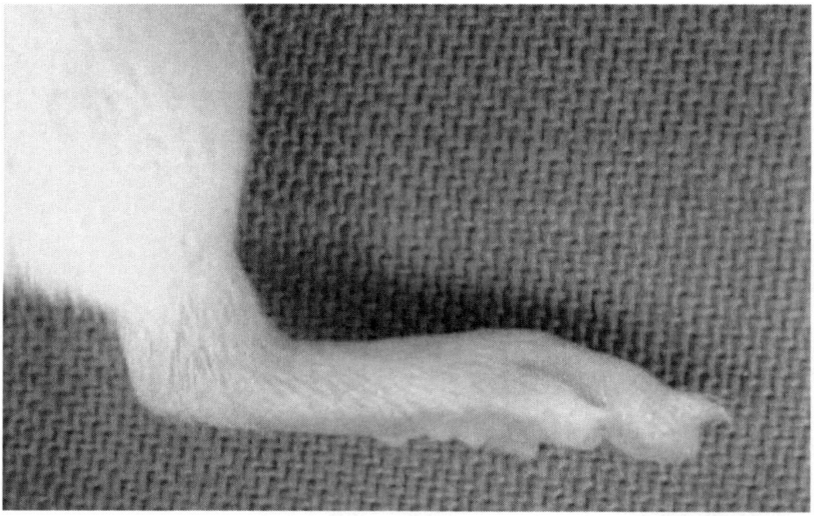

(B)

Figure 6. Representative macroscopic findings of the toenails of hemiplegia model mice. One month after denervation, the curvatures on the long axis of the third toenail of the denervated leg (A) and the innervated leg (B) were 87° and 100°, respectively.

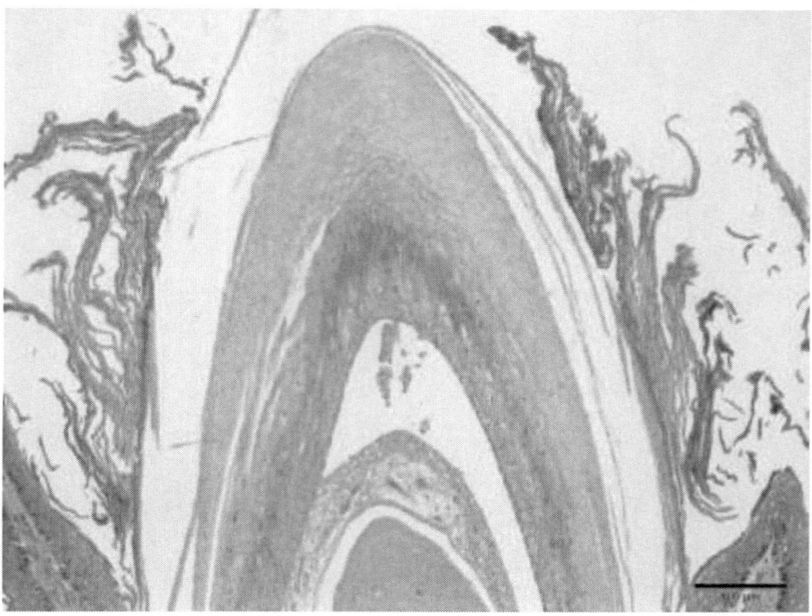

(A)

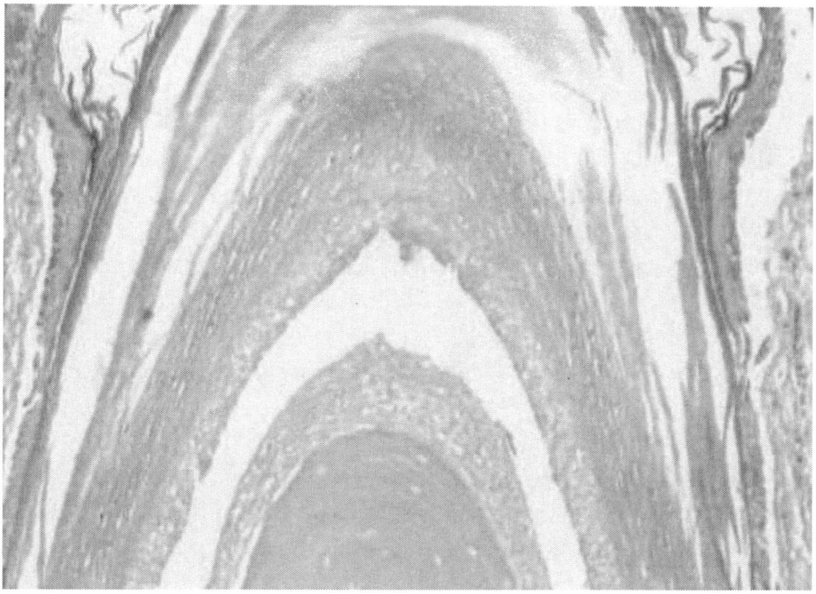

(B)

Figure 7. Representative microscopic findings of the third toenails of hemiplegia model mice. The nail curvatures on the short axis of the denervated leg (A) and the innervated leg (B) were 71° and 106°, respectively.

We hope that this review of the new concepts regarding nail deformities will help medical personnel and caregivers to understand the underlying mechanobiological processes that lead to these deformities. Mechanobiology-based studies that lead to the development of innovative methods that prevent and treat nail deformities are warranted.

REFERENCES

[1] Carter D. R., Beaupré G. S., Giori N. J., Helms J. A. Mechanobiology of skeletal regeneration. *Clin Orthop Relat Res.* 1998 Oct; (355 Suppl): S41-55.

[2] Sachs F., Sokabe M. Stretch-activated ion channels and membrane mechanics. *Neurosci Res Suppl.* 1990; 12:S1-4.

[3] Hayakawa K., Tatsumi H., Sokabe M. Actin stress fibers transmit and focus force to activate mechanosensitive channels. *J Cell Sci.* 2008 Feb 15; 121(Pt 4):496-503.

[4] Ingber D. E. Tensegrity and mechanotransduction. *J Body Mov Ther.* 2008 Jul; 12(3):198-200.

[5] Ingber D. E. Tensegrity-based mechanosensing from macro to micro. *Prog Biophys Mol Biol.* 2008 Jun-Jul; 97(2-3):163-79.

[6] 2008 marked the 150th anniversary of the publication of Gray's Anatomy, edited by Susan Standring, *Biomechanics of standing, walking and running,* chapter 84, 1459-1461.

[7] Abel M. F., Juhl G. A., Vaughan C. L., Damiano D. L., Gait assessment of fixed ankle-foot orthoses in children with spastic diplegia. *Arch Phys Med Rehabil* 1998; 79: 126-33.

[8] Brunner R., Meier G., Ruepp T. Comparison of a stiff and a spring-type ankle–foot orthosis to improve gait in spastic hemiplegic children. *J Pediatr Orthop* 1998; 18:719-26.

[9] Romkes J., Brunner R., Comparison of a dynamic and a hinged ankle-foot orthosis by gait analysis in patients with hemiplegic cerebral palsy. *Gait Posture* 2002; 15:18-24.

[10] J. Romkes, A. K. Hell, R. Brunner., Changes in muscle activity in children with hemiplegic cerebral palsy while walking with and without ankle-foot orthoses. *Gait & Posture* 24 (2006) 467-474.

[11] Hitomi Sano, Rei Ogawa, *Clinical evidence for the relationship between nail configuration and mechanical forces.* Plastic and Reconstructive Surgery - Global Open. In press.

[12] Hitomi Sano, Kaori Shionoya, Rei Ogawa, Finger Nail Configuration is Influenced by Mechanical Forces on Finger Pads. *J Dermatol.* 2013; 40(12):1056-7.

[13] Sano H., Ichioka S., Influence of mechanical forces as a part of nail configuration. *Dermatology* 2012; 225:210-214.

[14] Sano H., Shionoya K., Ogawa R., Impact of mechanical forces on finger nail curvature: an analysis of the impact of different occupations on 332 finger nails. *Dermatol Surg*2014; 40:441-445.

[15] Bentley, P. B. & Bayles M. A., Occupational koilonychia of the toe nails. *Br J Dermatol* 1971; 85: 140-144.

[16] Baran R., Haneke E., Richert B., Pincernails: Definition and surgical treatment. *Dermatol Surg* 2001; 27:261-6.

In: Paraplegia
Editor: Agnes A. Holloway
ISBN: 978-1-63482-465-1

Chapter 5

SPASTICITY

Win Min Oo, MD [*]
Physiatrist, Department of Physical Medicine and Rehabilitation,University of Medicine, Mandalay, Myanmar, Burma

ABSTRACT

Spasticity is characterized by a velocity-dependent increase in tonic stretch reflexes with exaggerated tendon jerks, resulting from hyperexcitability of the stretch reflex. It is a common complication affecting about 67% of the patients with spinal cord injury. Problematic spasticity occurs in 40-60% of these patients. When the injury is acute, muscle tone is flaccid with hyporeflexia (spinal shock) before the appearance of spasticity.

Muscle tone is maintained by regulation of stretch reflex arc which is balanced between the inhibitory influences by corticospinal tract and dorsal reticulospinal tract, and the facilitatory influences (on extensor tone) by medial reticulospinal and verstibulospinal tract (supraspinal control). Mechanism of spasticity is commonly explained by the combination of the following neurophysiological phenomena.

1) Presynaptic inhibition of Ia afferent terminals.
2) Disynaptic reciproval Ia inhibition from muscle spindle Ia afferents from the antagonist muscles.
3) Recurrent inhibition via Renshaw cells.

[*] E-mail: winminoo@ummdy.com; drwinminoopmr@gmail.com.

4) Non-reciprocal Ib inhibition from Golgi tendon organs.
5) Inhibition from muscle spindle group II afferents

Clinically, spasticity may be of different types due to involvement of different descending pathways. Depending on the predominant involvement of phasic (dynamic) or tonic (static) components of muscle stretch reflexes, the spasticity may be phasic or tonic. It can be separated into sub-definitions.

(1) Intrinsic tonic spasticity (manifesting as increased tone),
(2) Intrinsic phasic spasticity (manifesting as tendon hyper-reflexia and clonus) and
(3) Extrinsic spasticity manifesting as spasms

Spasticity is a clinical diagnosis. Measurement methods can be divided into clinical methods, biomechanical methods and electro-physiological methods. Spasticity is disabling and, if left untreated or sub-optimally treated, may lead to consequences, such as muscle shortening, contracture, limb deformity, altered body mechanics, loading on pressure points.

The successful management of spasticity can be a therapeutic challenge. Spasticity can assist weakened legs, permit transfer ability, and improve bed mobility. Therefore all spastic patients do not need treatments. It should be treated when it causes pain, difficulty in performing daily living activities, impaired mobility, poor joint positioning, increased risk of contracture, and skin breakdown.

The patient, caregiver, and healthcare professionals should agree about the treatment goals. The patient's age, preferences, and ability to comply with treatment need to be considered on the choice of treatment. The treatment of spasticity is usually initiated with the most conservative treatments that have the fewest risks. Treatment options include non-pharmacological, pharmacological and surgical interventions.

INTRODUCTION

The earliest reference to spinal cord injury (SCI) is found in the Edwin Smith Surgical Papyrus, written between 2500 and 3000 B.C as "an ailment not to be treated" (Kirshblum & Brooks, 2010).

It may cause paraplegia which involves the lower extremities or tetraplegia which involves all extremities, depending upon the level of injury (Cooper, 2006).

According to the American spinal injury association, it can be classified into two broad categories:

1) neurologically complete injury which does not have lowest sacral sparing and
2) neurologically incomplete injury which has lowest sacral sparing (Cooper, 2006).

DEFINITION OF SPASTICITY

Spasticity is defined as a motor disorder, characterized by a velocity-dependent increase in tonic stretch reflexes (muscle tone) with exaggerated tendon jerks, resulting from hyperexcitability of the stretch reflex (Lance, 1980).

In recent years, this definition has been challenged for two reasons. Firstly, many different clinical signs such as increased muscle tone, clonus, spasms and hyperreflexia are referred to as spasticity, but these symptoms can exist independently of each other and are not necessary to share a common pathophysiology (Nielsen et al., 2007).

Secondly, in several studies, many spastic patients on clinical examination did not have any signs of hyperreflexia (SchindlerIvens & Shields, 2004).

The increased muscle tone in such subjects seems to be caused by structural changes in the muscles (Dietz et al. 1981). Therefore, spasticity may also be explained by changes in muscle properties and not only by hyperreflexia and the altered central processing of sensory input in the spinal cord (Dietz et al., 1981, Gracies, 2005a,b).

However, it is difficult in distinguishing clinically between the increased hypertonia due to the passive muscular changes and that due to the stretch reflex changes. In such situation, it is useful to determine whether the muscle resistance is velocity -dependent or not. If the hypertonia is velocity-dependent, it would be a sign of spasticity and if not velocity-dependent, it would rather suggest muscular changes (Nielsen et al., 2007).

Epidermioogy of spasticity in SCI

Spasticity can accompany diffuse or localized cerebral or spinal pathology. Spasticity is often a significant problem in spinal cord injury (SCI), multiple sclerosis (MS), traumatic brain injury (TBI), cerebral palsy (CP), and stroke (Nance et al., 2011).

The 65–78% of chronic SCI patients have symptoms of spasticity (Adams & Hicks, 2005). Problematic spasticity is found in 40-60% of patients with SCI (Nance et al., 2011).

The ASIA classification of SCI (severity) and level of injury may predict the likelihood of developing spasticity. In individuals with cervical SCI, symptoms of spasticity occur in 93% of ASIA A patients and 78% of ASIA B–D patients. However, in individuals with thoracic SCI, spasticity is found in 72% of ASIA A patients and 73% of ASIA B–D patients (Skold et al., 1999).

Normal Regulation of the Motor Unit

Motor unit consists of an a motor neuron and all of the muscle fibers innervated by it. The control system requires such critical information as muscle length, velocity, muscle tension, and joint position. This is mediated by a combination of immediate monosynaptic reflexes and more complicated higher-level spinal and supraspinal polysynaptic activity. This activity can either facilitate or inhibit activity at the motor unit level. Units fire when the net excitation minus inhibition reaches their threshold (Elovic et al., 2010).

Motor Control by the Spinal Cord

Motor control by the spinal cord is basically dependent on the following factors.

1) Muscle Spindle and Monosynaptic Reflex

Physiology

This stretch reflex has two components: a brisk, short- acting phasic component and a weaker, longer-acting tonic component (Nance et al., 2011).

The intrafusal receptor organ (muscle spindle) detects changes in muscle length and contains three types of specialized fibers: dynamic nuclear bag fibers, static nuclear bag fibers and nuclear chain fibers.

Dynamic nuclear bag fibers are highly sensitive to the rate of change and provide phasic component of stretch reflex. Static nuclear bag fibers and nuclear chain fibers are more sensitive to the steady-state muscle length and gives tonic component of stretch reflex (Ganong et al., 2010).

Group Ia (primary sensory) afferents convey both phasic and tonic stretch information. Group II fibers convey only tonic stretch information from static nuclear bag and nuclear chain fibers. Gamma motor efferent fibers innervate the nuclear bag fibers and maintain spindle sensitivity during skeletal muscle contraction (Ganong et al., 2010).

During normal motor function, the gamma motor unit coactivates with the a motor neuron and maintains the spindle tension and efficiency (Elovic et al., 2010).

Significance

Muscle spindles geenerate muscle tone by acting through the stretch reflex. Tone is the constant muscular background activity that is necessary to maintain the basic attitude of the body particularly against the force of gravity (Carpenter, 1984).

As tone opposes movement and tends to keep muscles at preset lengths, it has to be changed in steps during a movement. Whenever a command is sent to alpha motor fibers, gamma fibers are also excited. So, alpha–gamma co-activation occurs to produce contraction of both extrafusal and intrafusal fibers according to the position and force commands from the brain to the spinal cord.

Clinical elicitation of stretch reflex is done in two ways:

a. Static – by passive stretching (tone testing).
b. Dynamic – by muscle and tendon jerks. (Mukherjee & Chakravarty, 2010)

2) Interneurons

They mediate most integrative functions in the spinal cord by involving in every segmental and stretch reflex pathways and being excited or inhibited by several peripheral and descending fiber systems (Lundberg, 1979).

As a consequence, spinal cord reflex responses are not stereotyped responses, but alters depending upon the ongoing activity in the surrounding interneurons (Davidoff, 1992)

The spinal interneurons play a critical role in normal motor control and spasticity. The effects of the Ia and Ib fibers are often mediated through Ia and Ib interneurons, respectively. The Renshaw cell and the propriospinal interneurons are also an important part of the control process (Elovic et al., 2010).

I) Ia Reciprocal Inhibition

Physiology

When the muscle contracts, the antagonist relaxes. The spindle impulses pass through a collateral of Ia afferent to the inhibitory neuron that synapses directly on the motor neuron of the antagonist muscles. This is bisynaptic and postsynaptic inhibition. Consequently, when the agonist muscle is excited, antagonists are inhibited simultaneously; a mechanism which is called reciprocal inhibition (Ganong et al., 2010).

Significance

la interneurons receive the same diverse excitatory and inhibitory inputs from segmental afferents (e.g., flexor afferents) and supraspinal descending tracts as alpha motoneurons do (Hultborn et al., 1976). These inputs excite alpha motoneurons to contract synergistic muscles and also excite la inhibitory interneurons to inhibit alpha motoneurons to antagonistic muscles during stretch reflex activity (Mukherjee & Chakravarty, 2010).

II) lb Non-reciprocal Inhibition

Physiology

The Golgi tendon organ is innervated by myelinated Ib sensory afferents. It is particularly sensitive to muscle tension created by active muscle contraction but has a high threshold for detecting passive stretch. Stimulation of Ib afferents results in inhibition of the homonymous α-motor neuron and of its synergists. This behavior has been called Ib non-reciprocal inhibition which is stimulated by muscle tension, whereas the stretch reflex is stimulated by a change in muscle length. (Nance et al., 2011) They serve to impose a ceiling effect on muscle contraction and prevent musculotendinous injury (Elovic et al., 2010).

Significance

Like la inhibitory interneurons, lb interneurons also receive diverse segmental and supraspinal inputs. Therefore, lb inhibition is not a simple autogenic inhibitory safety mechanism to regulate muscle tension only. It is a part of complex system regulating muscle tension to control posture and movement (Mukherjee & Chakravarty, 2010).

III) Recurrent Inhibition

Physiology

Renshaw cells are situated in lamina VII of ventral horn medial to motoneurons. Collateral from an alpha motoneuron axon excites Renshaw cell which in turn inhibits the same and other motoneuron innervating the synergistic muscles. This alpha motoneuron-Renshaw cell- α motoneuron pathway forms a negative feedback circuit to control motoneuron excitation and is called recurrent inhibition (Pompetano, 1984). In addition, Renshaw cells inhibit gamma motoneurons and la inhibitory interneurons (Jankowska & Roberts, 1972).

Significance

Renshaw cells inhibit the alpha motor neuron and its synergists in order to limit and stabilize the discharge frequency (Fleuren, 2009).

IV) Presynaptic Inhibition

Physiology

Inhibitory interneurons have presynaptic connections with la terminals and are under facilitatory supraspinal influences. Excitation of these interneurons reduces neurotransmitter release by 1a terminals on the alpha motor neurons, thereby maintaining a tonic inhibitory influence on the monosynaptic reflex arc, called presynaptic la inhibition (Fleuren, 2009).

Significance

The amplitude of EPSP in a motoneuron in response to la afferent stimulation decreases if there is prior depolarization of this la afferent fiber through axo-axonic synapse with a specific interneuron. Descending pathways control these specific interneurons involved in this process of presynaptic inhibition. This causes automatic suppression of unimportant afferent informations (Schmidt, 1971).

V) Flexor Reflex Afferents

Nociceptive reflex produces contraction of flexor muscles of a limb (withdrawal) and crossed extensor reflex of opposite limb. This is mediated by polysynaptic connection between flexor reflex afferents (FRA), interneurons and motoneurons of extensor as well as flexor muscles (Mukherjee & Chakravarty, 2010)

Reality is more complex, as the interneurons integrate afferent information of both la and lb afferents from various muscles and each interneuron forms widespread inhibitory synapses with both homonymous and heteronymous alpha motor neurons (Davidoff, 1992).

MOTOR CONTROL BY SUPRASPINAL INFLUENCES

Physiology

Supraspinal influences play a major role in both volitional movement and the pathophysiology of spasticity. Cortical lesions producing spasticity must involve both the primary motor and pre-motor cortices. Such lesions affect both pyramidal and parapyramidal cortico-reticular-spinal fibres (Sheean, 2008).

Supraspinal influences control spinal reflexes by converging on common interneuronal pool projecting to motoneurons. Imbalance of the descending inhibitory and facilitatory influences on muscle stretch reflexes is thought to be the cause of spasticity (Lundberg, 1975).

1) Inhibitory Supraspinal Pathways

There is an inhibitory area in the medullary reticular formation that is active as a powerful inhibitory center to regulate muscle tone (stretch reflex) and the cortical motor areas control tone through this center via cortico-reticular pathway. This medullary inhibitory centre gives off the dorsal reticulospinal tract (Sheean, 2008).

I) Corticoreticular Pathway

Isolated pyramidal lesions such as destruction of motor cortex (area 4) did not cause spasticity (Bucy et al., 1964). These lesions produced only weakness, hypotonia, hyporeflexia and Babinski's sign (Sheean, 2008). However, lesions of area 4 extending into the premotor and supplementary motor areas caused spasticity. Output fibers (cortico-reticular fibres) of these area run with the pyramidal tract, ending in the medullary reticular formation (Mukherjee & Chakravarty, 2010)

II) Dorsal Reticulospinal Tract

The output of the medullary inhibitory centre is the dorsal reticulospinal tract, which runs in the dorsolateral funiculus, adjacent to the lateral corticospinal (pyramidal) tract.

This tract is non-monoaminergic and inhibits FRA as well as stretch reflex arc. Flexor spams are release phenomenon of flexor reflexes due to damage to dorsal reticulospinal pathway (Fisher & Curry, 1965). Clasp-knife phenomenon is also a release phenomenon due to loss of inhibitory effects on FRA.

2) Excitatory Supraspinal Pathways

There are two areas forming the main excitatory system that facilitates spinal stretch reflexes and extensor tone.

I) Ventral Reticulospinal Tract

The tract has a diffuse origin being mainly from pontine tegmentum. It is not affected by stimulation of motor cortex or internal capsule and not inhibitory to FRA, which is unlike dorsal RST. Reticular formation exerts facilitatory influence on spasticity through this tract. This pathway is more important than vestibulospinal system in maintaining spastic extensor tone (Shahani & Young, 1973).

II) Vestibulospinal Pathway

It is a descending motor tract arising from lateral vestibular (Deiter's) nucleus. The tract ends mostly on interneurons but also excites motor neurons mono-synaptically. This excitatory pathway helps to support against gravity and so control extensors rather than flexors. This pathway is important in maintaining decerebrate rigidity but has lesser role in human spasticity (Fries et al., 1993).

Significance

The four descending pathways are arranged in the spinal cord as follows:

A) Lateral funiculus contains corticospinal tract and dorsal reticulospinal tract.
B) Anterior funiculus contains ventral reticulospinal tract and verstibulospinal tract (in close proximity with medial longitudinal fasciculus) as shown in the Fig. 6 (Sheean, 2008).

Mechanism of Spasticity

Dysfunction of descending pathways to and within the spinal cord gives rise to a UMN syndrome (Nance et al., 2011). It results from injury at cortical, brainstem, or spinal cord levels and spasticity evolves in the days and weeks after injury (Vanek, 2010).

Spinal Shock

When the injury is acute, muscle tone is flaccid with hyporeflexia before the appearance of spasticity (Vanek, 2010). Depressed spinal reflexes caudal to spinal cord injury (SCI) is defined as spinal shock. Ditunno et al. (2004) postulated a four-phase model of spinal shock, proposing possible mechanisms for each phase

When spinal shock is recovered, spasticity ensues. However, no single pathophysiologic mechanism can account for all the observable aspects of spasticity. Generally, spasticity develops when an imbalance occurs in the excitatory and inhibitory input to α motor neurons, resulting in hyperexcitability (Elovic et al., 2010).

Role of Spinal Excitatory Mechanisms in Spasticity

I) Increased Fusimotor Drive

Exaggerated muscle stretch reflexes in spasticity was once atributed the hyperactivity of γ- motoneurons that control the sensitivity of muscle spindles and stretch reflex gain. However, direct recordings from muscle spindles in SCI patients showed no increases in spindle activity during bouts of spasticity (Hagbarth et. al., 1973).

The prolonged duration for the development of spasticity after SCI suggests the contribution of plastic changes in other spinal pathways. Therefore, fusimotor hyperexcitability is unlikely to be involved in the pathophysiology of spasticity after SCI (Elbasiouny et al., 2010).

II) Denervation Hypersensitivity

Such hypersensitivity to neurotransmitters is occurs in the spinal cord as well as in the brain (Sawynok & Reid, 1994).

Proposed mechanisms include (1) reduced excitatory neurotransmitter reuptake, (2) increased synthesis and insertion of receptors into postsynaptic membrane, (3) decreased removal and degradation of receptor, and (4) altered synthesis and composition of receptor subunits. Upregulation in mRNA transcription and protein translation begins within hours and peaks in days. An increase in intracellular calcium associated with neuronal hypoactivity may lead to an increase in transcription–translation of receptors, channels, and growth factors (Ditunno et al., 2004).

III) Axonal Sprouting

McCouch et al. (1958) proposed another mechanism for spasticity. After SCI, terminals of the damaged axons on spinal neurons degenerate. By a few weeks post-injury, the remaining local afferents project new synaptic terminals in the vacated space and enhance the efficacy of the spinal connections. The prolongation of EPSP in spastic individuals supports the sprouting of Ia-afferents and the formation of new synapses on motoneurons. This mechanism could explain for the temporal changes in spasticity after SCI and the disruption in the balance between excitatory and inhibitory inputs to motoneurone. Thus, its significance to the pathophysiology of spasticity is high (Elbasiouny et. al., 2010).

IV) Primary Hyperexcitability of Alpha Motoneurons

In SCI patients with spasticity, an increase in the ratio of potentials resulting from electrical stimulation of the sensory and motor axons $_{(Hmax/Mmax)}$ was observed at rest (Delwaide, 1993). An increase in the amplitude and persistence of the F-wave was also found, further supporting the increased motoneuronal excitability (Hiersemenzel et al., 2000). This hyperexcitability was attributed to alterations in motoneuronal intrinsic properties, such as the activation of persistent inward currents (PICs) and depolarization of the membrane potential.

a) Persistent Inward Currents

A PIC is a depolarizing current that does not have inactivation with prolonged membrane depolarization. Normally, the motoneuronal PIC activation is controlled through the monoaminergic drive from the brainstem. After SCI, the PIC lost that control of descending drive, leading to uncontrolled and high motoneuronal firing rates with the results of the long-lasting exaggerated reflexes and muscle spasms (Elbasiouny et al., 2010).

In spinal motoneurons, PICs are mediated by 2 types of ion channels. After SCI, the Ca^{2+} PIC has little time-dependent inactivation and causes the long-lasting reflexes of spasticity whereas the Na+ PIC is partially inactivated with time and produce the spontaneous firing in association with a muscle spasm or voluntary contraction (Gorassini et al., 2004).

b) Differential Control of Spinal Neurons by Descending Drive

The monoaminergic drive from the brainstem control the excitability of spinal neurons during different motor tasks. This drive has differential effects on the ventral and dorsal horns of the spinal cord. In the ventral horn, monoamines have excitatory effects on motoneurons and low-threshold muscle afferents group I (Hammar et al., 2003).

In dorsal horn, monoamines hae inhibitory action on the motoneurone by presynaptic inhibition on the sensory inputs such as cutaneous and high-threshold muscle afferent inputs (groups III and IV). This differential control is due to the effect of different monoaminergic receptors. Motoneuronal facilitation acts through 5-HT_2 and NE a_1 receptors, whereas cutaneous and high-threshold muscle afferent inhibition is achieved through $_{5\text{-}HT1b/d}$ and NE a_2 receptors (Elbasiouny et al., 2010).

After SCI, this differential control changes. Acutely, the loss of the monoaminergic drive reduces the motoneuronal excitability in the ventral horn but increases EPSP of sensory inputs in the dorsal horn due to loss of inhibition. Despite the increased excitability of interneuronal pathways, long-lasting reflexes are not activated during this stage because of the reduced excitability of motoneurons. In the chronic stages of injury, motoneurons become highly sensitive to residual monoamines as a consequence of denervation hypersentivity. These facilitate the reactivation of the PICs and restore the motoneuronal excitability (Elbasiouny et al., 2010).

In this stage, prolonged EPSPs of sensory stimuli can activate the PIC and trigger long-lasting reflexes and muscle spasms. Thus, spasticity does not emerge until motoneurons become hyperexcitable, in spite of the increases in interneuronal excitability early after SCI. Therefore, the enhancement in motoneuronal excitability plays a significant role in the pathophysiology of spasticity (Elbasiouny et al., 2010).

V) Enhanced Excitability of Interneurons

The magnitude of flexor reflexes mediated by polysynaptic pathways was increased in individuals with spasticity after SCI (Hiersemenzel et al., 2000). Moreover, an increase in the ratio of excitatory-to-inhibitory inputs to motoneurons originating predominantly from spinal interneurons was observed during the development of spasticity. Therefore this mechanism plays a significant role in the pathophysiology of spasticity (Elbasiouny et al., 2010).

VI) Enhanced Cutaneous Reflexes

In spasticity, cutaneous reflexes (flexor or withdrawal) are increased. Dorsal horn neurons give rise to both long axons which form ascending tracts and short propriospinal axons to innervate motor neurons of cord. Rostral lesions in CNS disrupting the descending reticulospinal tract (RST) or spinothalamic tract alter normal gating mechanisms in dorsal horn so that pain is experienced to rather innocuous stimuli. Due to such mishandling of segmental inputs, hyperactivity in long tract neurons is felt as pain as an associated feature in spasticity (Mukherjee & Chakravarty, 2010)

Similarly excitation of short propriospinal interneuron system produces hyperactive nociceptive reflexes. This system acts as an arousal system for motoneurons in absence of brainstem reticular system due to SCI (Burke &

Ashby, 1972). The clinical signs of this phenomenon are Babinski's response, triple flexion of leg and gross flexor, or sometimes extensor spasm which may be produced by simple and non-noxious cutaneous stimuli (Mukherjee & Chakravarty, 2010).

ROLE OF SPINAL INHIBITORY MECHANISMS IN SPASTICITY

The monosynaptic Ia excitation which involves the dynamic and tonic components of the stretch reflex may be inhibited by various spinal reflexes pathways.

These include:

a) Presynaptic inhibition of Ia afferent terminals.
b) Disynaptic reciproval Ia inhibition from muscle spindle Ia afferents from the antagonist muscles.
c) Recurrent inhibition via Renshaw cells.
d) Non-reciprocal Ib inhibition from Golgi tendon organs.
e) Inhibition from muscle spindle group II afferents (Mukherjee & Chakravarty, 2010)

I) Presynaptic Inhibition of Ia Afferent Terminals

Presynaptic inhibition (PSI) controls the strength of synaptic inputs to neurons by regulating the levels of neurotransmitter release. Descending drives adjust PSI in a state-dependent manner. Loss of descending influenes causes a reduced presynaptic inhibition, resulting in the increased response on alpha motoneurons by Ia input and spasticity may occur (Mukherjee & Chakravarty, 2010).

In spastic SCI individuals, PSI evoked by muscle or tendon vibration at rest was reduced, which could result in the increased excitatability of Ia–motoneuron synapse (Faist et al., 1994).

The H-reflex disappeared during standing but was slightly depressed during walking relative to intact subjects. This altered modulation of reflexes during walking probably contributes to the stiff gait occuring after SCI (Yang et al., 1991). Thus, reduction in PSI is likely to be involved in the pathophysiology of spasticity following SCI. PSI has been the target of many antispastic drugs such as baclofen and benzodiazepines (Elbasiouny et al., 2010).

II) Disynaptic Reciprocal Ia Inhibition

In spastic patients, reflex spread is common with reflex- induced co-contraction of antagonist muscle groups. The Ia inhibitory interneurons are activated by descending motor fibers, damage to which could reduce this type of inhibition.

Regarding the nature of the alteration in Iareciprocal inhibition, different results were obtained. Boorman et al. (1996) showed that Ia reciprocal inhibition was reduced in individuals with spasticity after incomplete SCI. Crone et al. (2003) found that Ia- reciprocal inhibition was replaced by reciprocal excitation of antagonistic muscles after SCI, which facilitated co-contraction of antagonistic muscles during movements.

III) Recurrent Inhibition

In spastic patients due to spinal cord injury, increased rather than decreased recurrent inhibition may be seen (Shefner et al., 1992). However, increased recurrent inhibiton might contribute to spasticity by decreasing reciprocal Ia inhibition because Renshall cell inhibits the Ia afferent presynaptic inhibitory interneurone associated with the initiating motor neurone (Schomburg & Steffens, 1998).

IV) Non-reciprocal Ib Inhibition

Whereas this inhibition is easily demonstrated in healthy subjects, there was no inhibition on the paretic side in hemiplegic patients, along with a facilitatory effect in some subjects. Therefore, alteration of Ib inhibition excitation may plays a role in the pathophysiology of spasticity (Mukherjee & Chakravarty, 2010)

CLASSIFICATION OF SPASTICITY

Decq (2003) separated the components of spasticity into sub-definitions.

(1) Intrinsic tonic spasticity_ exaggeration of the tonic component of the stretch reflex (manifesting as increased tone),
(2) Intrinsic phasic spasticity_ exaggeration of the phasic component of the stretch reflex (manifesting as tendon hyper-reflexia and clonus) and
(3) Extrinsic spasticity – exaggeration of extrinsic flexion or extension spinal reflexes

INTRINSIC TONIC SPASTICITY

Decq (2003) defined it as the component of spasticity due to an exaggeration of the tonic component of the stretch reflex which results from a maintained stretch of the central region of the muscle fibers.

The hyperexcitability of this tonic stretch reflex cause the increased muscle tone in response to passive stretch (Sheean, 2008) and could be due to a lower threshold, an increased gain of the stretch reflex, or a combination of the two (Adams & Hicks, 2005).

Tonic stretch reflex can be dynamic, static or occur during active contraction (Sheean, 2008).

I) Dynamic Tonic Stretch Reflex

Spasticity results from velocity-sensitive hyperactive tonic stretch reflexes. In normal subjects, the reflex threshold was an angular velocity of around 200 degrees per second with the latency of the reflex being 61 to 107 ms, The reflex contraction was brief and was not maintained throughout the stretching movement (Rothwell, 1994).

In hemiparetic spastic (stroke) patients, Thilmann et al. (1991a) found that stretch reflexes could be elicited with relatively slow movements – as slow as 35 degrees per second. Reflex activity usually began at the end of the 61- to 107-ms latency window of normal subjects. However, it continued throughout the stretching movement and usually stopped just before the end of the displacement. The long latency of these reflexes suggests a polysynaptic pathway.

Burke et al. (1972) reported that the amount of reflex muscle contraction had a positive linear correlation with the velocity of stretch, supporting that spasticity is velocity-dependent.

Li et al. (2006) showed that tonic stretch reflexes (TSRs) are not only velocity-dependent but also length-dependent and there was an interaction between the two. Velocity dependence was greater at longer lengths and length dependence was greater with faster stretches. These observations marked the importance not only of velocity of stretch but also of body position and muscle length when measuring spasticity.

II) Static Tonic Stretch Reflexes

Thilmann et al., (1991a) found that there was no EMG activity, when the muscle was held in stretch the end of the movement. Thus, it has been considered that there is no appreciable static component to the tonic stretch reflex of spasticity.

However, several researchers have observed clear reflex activity in the maintained phase of a rampand-hold stretch of elbow flexors (Sheean, 2008)

The mechanism of static tonic stretch reflexes involves receptors that are chiefly sensitive to muscle length and less to velocity. The primary muscle spindles (with Ia afferents) are sensitive to both but mainly to velocity (Rothwell, 1994). The secondary muscle spindles, via the slower conducting group II afferents, maintain an increased firing level over baseline for as long as the muscle is held stretched (Sheean, 2008).

III) Tonic Stretch Reflexes during Muscle Activation

There is the modulation of stretch reflexes during more complex movements such as gait. In normal subjects, short-latency stretch reflexes of soleus show substantial phase-dependent modulation during walking, accounting as much as 30% to 60% of the soleus EMG activity during the stance phase. When supraspinal control was disrupted, this impairment of stretch reflex modulation contribute to the spastic gait disorder due to failure of the appropriate pattern of reflex suppression (Sheean, 2008).

IV) Nonreflex Contributions to Hypertonia

Neural hypertonia (spasticity) could lead to secondary biomechanical hypertonia such as fibrosis, atrophy of muscle fibers, decrease in the elastic properties, decrease in the number of sarcomeres, accumulation of connective tissue, and alteration of contractile properties toward tonic muscle characteristics (Adams & Hicks, 2005).

Such soft tissue changes can occur quite rapidly, as early as 2 months after stroke (Malouin et al., 1997). With appropriate timely intervention, these changes are reversible if the muscle is lengthened. However, prolonged immobilization at short length can result in irreversible shortening (Sheean, 2008).

Increased thixotropy could contribute to stiffness of the muscle fibres in spasticity. Thixotropy is a kind of resistance to muscle stretch due to cross-linking of actin and myosin filaments of muscle fibres and depends upon the history of the movement (Walsh, 1992). It also affects intrafusal fibres (primary muscle spindles), modifying their stretch sensitivity (Hagbarth et al., 1985).

Intrinsic Phasic Spasticity

Intrinsic phasic spasticity is due to exaggeration of the phasic component of the stretch reflex and includes tendon hyper-reflexia and clonus (Decq, 2003).

I) Tendon Hyper-Reflexia

Tendon hyper-reflexia is an exaggerated muscle response to an externally applied tap of deep tendons. It was assumed that the occurrence of reduced presynaptic inhibition of group Ia fibers would correlate with the excitability of tendon reflexes (Adams and Hicks, 2005).

However, of the two studies on tizanidine which was proved to reduce presynaptic inhibition, clonus was reduced in one study (Delwaide & Pennisi, 1994), but tendon reflexes were unchanged in another (Milanov & Georgiev, 1994). This discrepancy challenged the earlier conclusion that impaired presynaptic inhibition correlates better with tendon hyperreflexia than with muscle hypertonia.

In the UMN syndrome, percussion of one tendon often produces similar brief reflex contractions of other muscles in the limb, a phenomenon known as reflex irradiation. Mechanism is that tendon percussion sets up a wave of vibration through the limb that is capable of exciting spindles in other muscles, evoking phasic stretch reflexes if the stretch reflexes of those muscles are also hyperexcitable (Sheean, 2008).

II) Clonus

Clonus is involuntary rhythmic muscle contraction, menifesting as distal joint oscillation (Rossi et al., 1990). Clinically, ankle clonus is elicited through a quick and maintained stretch of the ankle plantarflexors that results in prolonged ankle oscillation. In patients with SCI, severe clonus can interrupt sleep, hinder transferring capabilities, and cause fatigue to the point of detracting from job performance. In addition, the inability of some patients to stand or walk independently has been attributed to severe clonus (Beres-Jones et al., 2003).

There were two theories for clonus mechanism. The first theory is that the clonus is due to the recurrent activation of stretch reflexes (Rossi et al., 1990). Dorsiflexing the ankle activates the Ia muscle spindle afferents and causes a reflex contraction of the triceps surae, plantar flexing the ankle, which is brief. The muscle then relaxes, causing the ankle to be dorsiflexed once again due to the sustained stretch of an examiner. The result is a new stretch reflex and it is called the sustained clonus (Beres-Jones et al., 2003).

The second theory is that clonus is the result of activity of a central oscillator or generator within the spinal cord, which rhythmically activates alpha motor neurons in response to peripheral events. Beres-Jones et al. (2003) supported such a hypothesis because of (1) reports that clonus frequencies among ankle, knee, and wrist muscles were similar, (2) the fact that the input frequency did not entrain the clonus, suggesting the clonus was not solely stretch-mediated (3) the finding that stimuli other than stretch evoke clonus, and (4) the observation of a refractory period following the clonic EMG burst where tendon tap, H-reflex stimulation, and vibration fail to elicit an efferent response.

In addition, Beres-Jones et al. (2003) obtained the following conclusion from their experiment.

1) Recurrent stretch reflex cannot be the sole mechanism of clonus because they found that clonic EMG in the SOL, MG, and TA occurred while the ankle was held isometrically in plantarflexion. In addition, SOL, MG, and TA activation occurred synchronously with similar burst durations, silent periods, and frequencies during plantarflexor stretch-induced ankle clonus
2) Peripheral events interacting with centrally mediated networks induce clonus. The clonic EMG occurred over a wide range of kinematic and kinetic conditions and thus proprioceptive inputs. However, clonus can occur at a stable frequency, independent of changes in peripheral events that modulate muscle lengthening and loading They cited that Dimitrijevic et al. (1980) reported that clonus frequency re mained constant with differing tendon tap frequencies.
3) Clonic EMG occurred with similar frequencies during both the stance and swing phases of the step cycle, occurring not only when load was applied to the limb, but also when there was no background force to maintain stretch, strongly supporting that neurons within the spinal cord with oscillatory properties can be activated by a myriad of afferent events.

They concluded that the synchronous oscillatory motor output may be a reorganization of neural networks in response to chronically altered afferent and supraspinal inputs (Beres-Jones et al.' 2003).

EXTRINSIC SPASTICITY

Involuntary muscle spasms can occur in response to a noxious stimulus coming from extrinsic to the muscle (Decq, 2003). Flexion spasms are the most common form, triggered by flexor reflex afferents from skin, muscle, subcutaneous tissues, and joints, which mediate the flexion withdrawal reflex (Sheean, 2008). SCI can interrupt the inhibition of these reflexes by supraspinal pathways, making them hyperexcitable (Decq, 2003). Plateau potentials in the spinal interneuronal and motoneuronal circuitry implicates in this mechanism. Intrasegmental poly-synaptic connections cause the flexor reflex initiated by a localized stimulus to generate a widespread flexor spasm, menifesting as a coordinated flexion of all joints of the leg (Adams & Hicks, 2005).

Differences between Cerebral and Spinal Spasticity

The pattern of spasticity due to cerebral lesions is somewhat different to that of spinal lesions. With cerebral lesions, spasticity can be less severe and more often involve the extensors with a posture of lower limb extension. Flexor spasms are rare and the clasp-knife phenomenon is uncommon. Clonus tends also to be less severe.

In contrast, spinal lesions can have very severe spasticity, more often in flexors with a dominant posture of lower limb flexion (paraplegia in flexion). Flexor spasms and clasp-knife phenomenon are more common, as is clonus.

The pathophysiological reasons for these differences depend on three factors.

1) The cortico-reticular fibres drive the inhibitory brainstem centre,
2) The inhibitory and excitatory tracts are separate anatomically in the spinal cord
3) Both the excitatory and inhibitory systems inhibit flexor reflex afferents, which are responsible for flexor spasms.

A suprabulbar lesion would lose its cortical facilitation over the inhibitory brainstem centre. However, this inhibitory centre could continue to contribute some inhibition of spinal stretch reflexes and flexor reflex afferents but with a partial reduction in inhibitory drive. And so, the excitatory system would still dominate, facilitating extensors while also inhibiting flexor reflex afferents. Hence, the spasticity would be milder in form and more extensor in type with fewer flexor spasms than spinal spasticity (Sheean, 2008).

Diagnosis

Spasticity is a clinical diagnosis. Assessment of spasticity includes identification of which muscles or muscle groups are overactive and determination of the spasticity effect on all aspects of patient function such as activities of daily living (ADLs), mobility and employment.

PRECIPITATING FACTORS

These factors can be divided into external and internal stimuli as in the following Table 1.

Table 1. Peripheral causes of aggravated muscle over activity

External stimuli	Internal stimuli
• Tight clothing • Tight bandages, orthoses, etc. • Kinked/blocked catheters • Condom drainage • appliances	• Constipation, especially colonic faecal loading • Infection and abscesses • Urinary retention and • Infection • Pressure sores • Heterotopic ossification • Fractures/dislocations

SPASTICITY OF THE LOWER EXTREMITIES

Spastic deformities of the lower limbs affect ambulation, bed positioning, sitting, chair level activities, transfer and standing up.

In the flexed knee, over-activity in the hamstrings is more often medial than lateral. Adductor and hip flexors spasticity often coexist and may lead to pelvic obliquity (Vanek, 2010).

The pes equinus(plantarfleion) is a key deformity that can interfere with functional ambulation or unassisted transfer (Vanek, 2010).

In spasticity of SCI patients, plantar flexion of the ankle during gait is a common finding, resulting from a combination of overactivity of the plantar flexors due to spasticity and underactivity of the ankle dorsiflexors The latter was attributed to the weakness from the UMN lesion and possibly reciprocal inhibition by the presumed overactive plantarflexors. Therefore, spasticity could play a role in the gait disturbance (Sheean, 2008).

In addition to gait disturbance, it can compromise walking stbility and often results in decreased stride length and walking speed. It can create balance difficulties and increase energy demands (Neptune et al., 2007).

A pes equinus position, while walking and certainly in case of first contact of the foot with the ground in early stance phase, is often called toe-walking. In upper motor neurone syndrome, it is position and motion-dependent; the symptoms of abnormal muscle contraction depend on the position (lying, sitting position) and motion (walking, running). These symptoms therefore increase from lying to sitting to standing, while walking and most of all while running (if possible).

Patients with a spastic paresis have a different way of walking. The following types of gait can be identified:

1. Gait characterised by drop foot
2. Gait characterised by (hyper) extension of the knee in the mid-stance phase
3. Gait characterised by hyperextension of the knee in mid-stance phase without heel contact
4. Gait characterised by flexion of the knee in mid-stance phase without heel contact
5. Gait characterised by flexion of the knee in mid-stance phase with full foot contact (Neptune et al., 2007)

Assessment of Severity

No standard measure is available for spasticity and outcome of its treatment. Therefore Malhotra et al. (2009) titled spasticity as "an impairment that is poorly defined and poorly measured".

Measurement methods for spasticity can be divided into clinical methods, biomechanical methods and electrophysiological methods.

Clinical Methods

The most often used in the clinical settings is the Modified Ashworth Scale due to easy availability and less time-consumption.

I) Ashworth Measure of Spasticity

The Ashworth measure of spasticity was developed as a simple clinical classification of spasticity (Ashworth, 1964). It is a five-point nominal scale focusing on the subjective clinical assessment of tone (Table 2). For the MAS, an additional grade was added (1+) to enhance sensitivity (Bohannon & Smith, 1987). These measures have been adopted for assessing spasticity in various indications including SCI although characteristics of spasticity are not the same in different etiologies.

Table 2. The Ashworth and modified Ashworth scales

Ashworth Scale	Score	Modified Ashworth Scale
No increase in tone	0	No increase in tone
Slight increase in tone giving a 'catch' when the limb was moved in flexion or extension	1	Slight increase in muscle tone, manifested by a catch and release or by minimal resistance at the end range of motion when the affected part(s) is moved in flexion or extension
	1+	Slight increase in muscle tone, manifested by a catch, followed by minimal resistance throughout the remainder (less than half) of the ROM
More marked increase in tone but limb easily flexed	2	More marked increase in muscle tone through most of the ROM, but the affected part(s) is easily moved
Considerable increase in tone – passive movement difficult	3	Considerable increase in muscle tone, passive movement is difficult
Limb rigid in flexion or extension	4	Affected part(s) rigid in flexion or extension

The scale determines the amount of resistance felt during the passive displacement of a limb, but it does not account accurately for the dependence of the resistance to the velocity of the stretch (Steeves et al., 2007). For AS, inter-rater reliability is adequate for specific lower limb muscles, such as the adductors and flexors but poor for the plantar flexors (Hsieh et al., 2008).

The AS correlates most strongly with the patellar tendon tap (Priebe et al., 1996). Sherwood et al. (2000) found correlations of the AS and MAS with EMG and suggested that AS does not discriminate well at the low end of spasticity (AS score 0 vs 1).

The AS and MAS are simple to administer, are well tolerated, require no specialized equipment, but only address the velocity-dependent aspect of spasticity across a single joint(Hsieh et al., 2008).

The AS and MAS were the spasticity outcome measures most commonly used and psychometrically assessed in SCI. Target muscle group and severity of spasticity should be considerations in the selection between AS and MAS. Validity for both AS and MAS has only been partially established and even less so for responsiveness (Hsieh et al., 2008).

II) Penn Spasm Frequency Scale

Penn et al. (1989) originally defined a five-point spasm frequency scale, which was later modified by Priebe et al. (1996)) and referred to as the modified PSFS (Table. 3). The modified PSFS is a two-component self-report scale to improve clinical ratings of spasticity.

Table 3. Penn spasm frequency scale and the spasm frequency score

Penn spasm frequency scale	score	spasm frequency score
No spasms	0	No spasms
Mild spasms at stimulation	1	One or fewer spasms per day
Irregular strong spasms less than 1 time/h	2	Between 1 and 5 spasms per day
Spasms more often than 1 time/h	3	Five to less than 10 spasms per day
Spasms more than 10 times/h	4	Ten or more spasms per day, or continuous contraction

The first component is a five-point scale assessing the frequency with which spasms occur. The second component is a three-point scale assessing the severity of spasms ranging from '1 = mild' to '3 = severe'. This measure is simple and appropriate to the clinical setting and does not require specialized equipment to perform (Hsieh et al., 2008).

Reliability has not been established for PSFS in SCI. By utilizing a standard time specification for the self-report, the 'present' spasm severity self-report correlated modestly to AS, whereas the 'in general' spasm severity self-report correlated poorly to AS (Hsieh et al., 2008).

Table 4. The quality of the muscle reactions (X) when using the Tardieu scale

Grade	Quality of muscle reaction
0	No resistance throughout the course of the passive movement
1	Slight resistance throughout the course of the passive movement, with no clear catch at precise angle
2	Clear catch at precise angle, interrupting the passive movement, followed by release
3	Fatiguable clonus (<10 seconds when maintaining pressure) occurring at precise angle
4	Infatiguable clonus (>10 seconds when maintaining pressure) occurring at precise angle

III) Tardieu Scale

The angle at the point of resistance is noted by stretching a limb passively. This is performed during as slow a movement as possible (V1), under gravitational pull (V2) and at a fast rate (V3). The examiner will feel a catch in a muscle under the influence of an overactive stretch reflex. Five levels have been described at the point of this catch to capture the quality of the muscular reaction (Table 4). In essence the scale assesses dynamic and static muscle length as well as joint range of motion (Bandi & Ward, 2010).

The inter and intra-rater reliability is generally good but the technique does require training to achieve this (Bandi & Ward, 2010).

IV) Composite Spasticity Score

The clinical score which is often used in research is composite spasticity score (annex II). It includes three scales: 5-point Achilles tendon jerks, double-weighted 5-point Asworth scale and 4-point ankle clonus.

This is also called global spasticity score because it can give extra information on the phasic component of the stretch reflexes due to inclusion of tendon jerks and clonus in addition to the static component. The scores ranging from 1-5, 6-9, 10-12, 13-16 correspond to normal, mild, moderate and severe spasticity (Nadeau et al., 1999).

Levin and Hui-Chan (1992) had established the test-retest reliability in rating the spasticity in hemiplegic patients (intraclass correlation coefficient = 0.87).

Nadeau et al. (1999) made a trial to assess this score in chronic stroke and SCI patients and concluded that it was a relevant clinical tool for assessment in muscle tone of lower limb in different neurologic population.

Nielsen and Sinkjaer (1996) made a spasticity assessment trial in multiple sclerosis cases. They reported that biomechanical and electrophysiological evaluation of spasticity at the ankle joint was related to the over-all total muscle tone and reflex scores of lower extremities.

There are many trials which used composite spasticity scale in upper motor neuron lesions such in MS, CP, SCI and stroke.

Miller et al. (2007) used CSS as outcome measure in a trial of TENS in MS, Shamay and Hui-Chan (2009) in stroke and Oo WM (2014) in subacute SCI.

The other measures are the Bilateral Adductor Tone Score, and the Visual Analog Scale (Elovic & Baerga, 2004).

Biomechanical Methods

I) Wartenberg Pendulum Test

The pendulum test was introduced by Wartenberg (1951). In its most simple form, the patient is seated or lying with the lower leg hanging over the end of a couch. The knee is released from full extension and the leg is allowed to swing freely under the action of gravity until motion ceased. In normal person, the leg would swing about six times after release and it was proposed to assess the severity of spasticity by counting the number of swings (Johnson and Pandyan, 2008).

Using electrogoniometers, Bajd and vodovnik (1984) proposed the relaxation index, based on the rate of decay of oscillation as a quantitative measure of spasticity. This index shows a clear correlation to the AS (Biering-Sørensen et al., 2006).

The advantage of the pendulum test is its simplicity. However, it also has several drawbacks. It may only be used to evaluate spasticity in the knee muscles and it seems not useful in severe spasticity. This test might not distinguish increased resistance in the muscle due to viscoelastic changes from the velocity-dependent resistance due to spasticity. And so, the test has not obtained any wider use (Biering-Sørensen et al., 2006).

II) Isokinetic Dynamometers

Isokinetic dynamometers have frequently been used for evaluation of spasticity. These devices can make a standardization of the applied stretch velocity and amplitude and so quantification of the velocity-dependent resistance of the muscle to passive movement.

They may be useful when an objective and reproducible spasticity measure is needed, such as research projects and drug evaluation. They can also determine the velocity-dependency of the muscle resistance, contributions from intrinsic muscle resistance and stretch-evoked muscle resistance (Biering-Sørensen et al., 2006).

Electrophysiological Methods

Several studies during the past 40–50 years have used EMG to evaluate its relatioship to the degree of spasticity (Biering-Sørensen et al., 2006).

I) H Reflexes

The H reflex is a long-latency reflex obtained by submaximally stimulating the Ia afferent pathways in a mixed nerve It was used to study both excitability in the Ia afferent pathways and abnormalities in presynaptic and reciprocal inhibition (Rothwell, 1994).

However, different outcomes may result from variations in stimulus intensity, the resting posture of the limb, the ability of a subject to relax or the neck and vestibular reflexes, and the results should be treated with caution. In order to normalize for this variability, the H-reflex response has been expressed as a percentage of the M-response (i.e., the stimulus of a muscle to supramaximal stimulation). However, the correlation between H/M ratios and the severity of spastic hyperreflexia was poor (Voerman et al., 2005).

II) F waves

F waves are obtained by the supramaximal stimulation of a mixed nerve and have been used as a measure of a-motor neurone excitability. The average F-wave response from repeated tests is often used because of variations in latency and amplitude. The spastic subjects show increased F-wave amplitudes, suggesting increased motor neuronal excitability (Voerman et al., 2005).

However, more research is still required to develop this as a reliable clinical measure of spasticity. The primary problem with existing electrophysiological methods seem to be the poor correlation with the other clinical techniques (Johnson & Pandyan, 2008).

Complications of Spasticity

Spasticity is disabling and, if left untreated or sub-optimally treated, may lead to consequences, such as:

- muscle shortening
- contractures (leading to abnormal body segment loading and sensory change)
- limb deformity and altered body mechanics, altered body image
- the need for special wheelchairs and seating and pressure-relieving equipment
- loading on pressure points
- pressure sores
- difficulty in the management of pressure sores
- pain from muscle spasms
- degenerative joint disease

- loss of function and
- mood problems and inability to participate in rehabilitation.

Painful spasms and tendon traction on bones is well known and the complications will prevent patients from achieving their optimal functioning. Deconditioning from ill-health and pain will also have a negative effect and cause reduced quality of life. There are therefore very good clinical, humanistic and economic reasons to treat it effectively and judiciously (Bandi & Ward, 2010).

Although associated with complications, spasticity is beneficial to some patients. It may help to transfer, stand and ambulate, maintain muscle bulk, prevent deep vein thrombosis and osteoporosis (Bandi & Ward, 2010).

Management

The successful management of spasticity can be a therapeutic challenge. Spasticity can assist weakened legs, permit transfer ability, and improve bed mobility.Therefore all spastic patients do not need treatments. It should be treated when it causes pain, difficulty in performing daily living activities, impaired mobility, poor joint positioning, increased risk of contracture and skin breakdown (Nance et al., 2011).

The patient, caregiver, and healthcare professionals should agree about the treatment goals. The patient's age, preferences, and ability to comply with treatment need to be considered on the choice of treatment.

The treatment of spasticity is usually initiated with the most conservative treatments that have the fewest risks. Treatment options include non-pharmacological, pharmacological and surgical interventions.

Non-pharmacological Management

A regular exercise routine and a high index of suspicion for spasticity and its triggering factors (e.g., urinary tract infection, constipation, ingrown nails and etc.) are the mainstays for preventing the change from the simple presence of spasticity to that of spasticity causing loss of function (Nance et al., 2011).

I) Education

When utilizing any first line rehabilitation strategies in the management of spasticity, interventions must carry over into a person's daily routine. Adherence to home exercise programs is crucial. Education encourges patients to make informed decisions regarding their healthcare and fosters investment in their own treatment plans, and also facilitates active participation in the ongoing treatment process (Bandi & Ward, 2010).

II) Physiotherapy

Whereas antispastic drugs act on the neural component of spasticity, physiotherapy minimizes the biomechanical side effects. Increased muscle tone causes spastic muscles to resist stretch and remain shortened for long durations, which leads to joint deformity and changes in the intrinsic properties of soft tissues and muscle fibers. This in turn restricts the range of motion and decrease the functional use of residual voluntary movements in patients with incomplete SCI. These changes contribute a biomechanical component to spasticity (Elbasiouny et al., 2010).

a) Positioning and Seating

Poor positioning can cause the increase in spasticity and the decrease in range of motion which leads to contractures, the noxious stimulation, pain, and exacerbation of a vicious cycle that can result in worsening spasticity (Elovic et al., 2010).

Therefore, correct positioning is an essential stage of management, especially for the immobile patient. Incorrect positioning in bed is a major cause of unnecessary spasticity. The supine position easily exacerbate extensor spasm by facilitation of the tonic labyrinthine supine reflex in stroke patients. Similarly, a number of patients exhibit an asymmetric tonic neck reflex after brain injury which will encourage a windswept posture in the supine position. Side lying, sitting and standing can all be helpful in different circumstances in order to reduce spasticity and produce stretch on the spastic muscles, as well as facilitate the use of antagonistic muscle groups (Barnes, 1998).

The spasticity can be exacerbated by a scissoring position (bilateral hip extension, adduction, internal rotation) and windswept position (hip flexion, abduction, external rotation on one side and relative hip extension, adduction, and internal rotation on the other), which should be avoided (Elovic et al., 2010).

Proper seating is vital. The body should be contained in a balanced, symmetrical and stable posture which is both comfortable and maximizes function. The pelvis should be stablized without lateral tilt or rotation, but with a slight anterior tilt so the spine adopts a normal lumbar lordosis, thoracic kyphosis and cervical lordosis. The hip should be maintained at an angle of slightly more than 90°, which is often facilitated by a seat cushion with a slight backward slope. Knees and ankles should be at 90^0 (Barnes, 1998).

In people with severe spasticity, this posture may not be possible or may require a variety of seating adjustments such as foot straps, knee blocks, adductor pommels, lumbar supports, lateral trunk supports and a variety of head and neck support systems. An adaptable and adjustable system is useful, particularly in people with complicated disabilities (Barnes, 1998).

b) Range of Motion Exercise

Range of motion exercise is necessary for maintaining optimum joint mobility and minimizing the risk of joint contracture. The spastic persons have far grater risk of complications due to muscle and joint tightness and impaired range of motion than those without. It should be initiated as early as possible (Bandi & Ward, 2010).

Each joint should be put through a full range of movement for at least 2 h in everyday (Barnes, 1998).

c) Stretching

Stretching is crucial in minimizing the risk for muscle shortening due to spasticity. Shortening of the soft tissues inevitably results in decreased range of motion, and may result in pain and loss of function (increased disability). It may be efficient to focus on commonly shortened muscles (e.g., iliopsoas which may contribute to low back pain and gait disorders), and biceps (which may limit coordinated upper extremity function) and those muscles that cross two joints (e.g., rectus femoris, and gastrocnemius).

For optimal effect, stretching must be performed daily. A stretch must be sustained in order to reduce spasticity; some suggest holding a stretch for >1 minute, while others suggest a prolonged stretch (hours) by using a splint or a brace (Bandi & Ward, 2010).

It should be performed at least two or three times per day as part of any treatment regime for spasticity (Bavikatte & Gaber, 2009).

When the patient is paralyzed as in SCI, passive stretching exercises decrease the complication of immobilization, minimizes the effects of formation of contracture, maintains the mechanical elasticity of muscles, causes temporary reduction in intensity of muscle contraction in reaction to muscle stretch, leads to plastic changes within the central nervous system and/or mechanical changes at the muscle, tendon, and soft-tissue level (Nance, 2003).

At least partial maintenance of reduced spasticity with a VAS question was noted when patients are asked to rate spasticity from "none" to "worst imaginable" on the 4 th day after the last treatment session (Hsieh et al., 2007).

d) Strengthening

There is a risk of progressive weakening of spastic muscles due to inactivity. As a result, it is important that strengthening programs are initiated early, and that strength in spastic muscles is optimized. There is no existing literature to suggest one form of strengthening exercise over another (Bandi & Ward, 2010).

e) Massage

Although various techniques are in use, there is no evidence to support this (Bandi & Ward, 2010).

f) Dynamic Physiotherapy Technique

There are a number of different dynamic physiotherapy techniques, including the Bobath technique, proprioceptive neuromuscular facilitation, the Brunnstrom technique and the techniques proposed by Carr and Shepherd (Barnes, 1998).

All claim to have antispastic and functional benefits, particularly for the more mobile person (Bandi & Ward, 2010).

g) Splinting and Casting

A splint is an external device designed to apply, distribute or remove forces to or from the body in a controlled manner to control body motions and /or alter the shape of body tissues, e.g., ankle foot orthosis. Some equipment can also aid positioning e.g., T roles, wedges, cushions and foot straps (Bandi & Ward, 2010).

The application of splints and casts can prevent the formation of contractures in the spastic limb and serial casting can improve the range of movement in a joint that is already contracted. It is uncertain about whether this is purely a mechanical effect or whether splinting actually reduces spasticity. However, there is no clear agreement on the most appropriate design nor the length of application time for a splint to give the desired effect (Barnes, 1998).

Ankle Foot Orthoses (AFO)

AFOs aid in gait by controlling the equinus or equino varus deformity.

Tone Reducing AFOs

They have certain features designed to decrease abnormal reflexes, including a foot plate that extends past the toe to discourage toe flexion and a metatarsal support to discourage stimulation to a particularly reflexogenic area of the foot. They are most effective during gait, but use during rest helps prevent contractures (Elovic and Baerga, 2004).

These are usually used in combination with other modalities like botox therapy. Attention to posture and positioning is paramount in managing severe spasticity (Bandi & Ward, 2010).

III) Physical Modalities

a) Cooling of Muscles

This inhibits monosynaptic stretch reflex and lowers the receptor's sensitivity. Different techniques such as quick icing and evaporating spray like ethyl chloride are occasionally used (Bandi & Ward, 2010).

b) Heat

Heat may increase the elasticity of the muscles. Techniques used include ultrasound, fluidotherapy, paraffin, superficial heat and whirlpools. These techniques should be combined with stretching and exercise (Bandi & Ward, 2010).

c) Electrical Stimulation

Various electrical stimulation modalities have been used to reduce the level of spasticity. There are four main types of electrical stimulation.

1) Neuromuscular electrical stimulation,
2) Threshold or therapeutic electrical stimulation
3) Functional electrical stimulation

4) Transcutaneous electrical stimulation

1) Neuromuscular Electrical Stimulation (NMES)

It provides functional re-education by directly causing an active muscle contraction. Surface electrodes are applied to the skin over motor points to depolarize the nerve to a specific muscle or muscles. It is used for short periods of time in combination with exercises. The overall goal is to strengthen the targeted muscles and to increase the functional use of this muscle (Patel, 2005).

A single application of neuromuscular electrical stimulation reduced spasticity immediately although these effects waned and were mostly absent by the next day. Spasticity reduction was seen in torque resistance to sinusoidal ankle movement, pendulum test, and MAS but not clonus scores or Hreflexes. These findings provide level 2 evidence for the role of neuromuscular electrical stimulation in reducing spasticity (Hsieh et al., 2007).

2) Threshold or Therapeutic Electrical Stimulation (TES)

It is a low-level electrical stimulation. It does not elicit actual muscle contraction; rather it causes just a comfortable tingling sensation. Surface electrodes are applied over the muscle. It is used for 8-12 hour periods of time during sleep. It is believed to increase the muscle blood flow and bulk (Patel, 2005).

3) Functional Electrical Stimulation (FES)

It is the application of electrical stimulation during a given task or activity when a specific muscle is expected to be contracting. Specifically, it can support the restoration of mobility in paralyzed individuals. The goal is to produce movements or functions which mimic normal voluntary activity (Patel, 2005).

4) Transcutaneous Electrical Nerve Stimulation (TENS)

It is used in treatment sessions and/or at home for the primary concern of temporary pain relief. Lately, it has been used to reduce spasticity. There are three main types of TENS, which are conventional TENS, acupuncture-like TENS and burst TENS (Walsh and Basford, 2009).

Han et al. (1994) treated thirty-two spastic SCI patients with a transcutaneous electrical nerve stimulator, the Han's acupoint nerve stimulator (HANS) via skin electrodes placed over the acupoints on the hand and leg. Their study showed that high frequency (100 Hz), but not the low frequency (2

Hz), stimulation was effective in reducing muscle spasticity. While the therapeutic effect lasted for only 10 minutes in the first treatment, it became consolidated after consecutive daily treatment for 3 months. The anti-spastic effect induced by high frequency electrical stimulation can be partially reversed by a high dose of naloxone. They discussed that the anti-spastic effect is mediated, at least in part, by the endogenous opioid ligand interacting with the kappa opiate receptors, most probably dynorphin, in the central nervous system.

Goulet et al. (1996) examined the short-term effects of TENS with electrical parameters of 99 Hz; 0.25 msec pulses and an intensity of 15 mA on H-reflex and clinical spasticity in fourteen SCI patients. They hypothesized that repetitive low-threshold afferent electrical stimulation would have an inhibitory effect on the triceps surae H-reflexes and plantar flexor spasticity. They measured ankle clonus, Achilles tendon reflex and Modified Ashworth scale before and after a 30-minutes application of TENS. These tests failed to reveal any significant effects of TENS on H-reflex amplitude in patients with spinal cord injuries. However, there was a significant decrease in scores for the Achilles tendon reflex and the Modified Ashworth test. The clonus scores also decreased in most patients post-TENS but not significantly. The results thus suggested that TENS appears to be effective in reducing spinal spasticity clinically. Moreover, the absence of significant effects of TENS on H-reflex amplitude, despite a significant reduction in the clinical spasticity score, might reflect that repetitive stimulation of the low-threshold afferent influenced on the sensitivity of the spinal receptors that are bypassed for the elicitation of of the H-reflex.

Gregoric (1998) studied the effects of the transcutaneous electrical nerve stimulation (TENS) to the area of the sural nerve on the early and late electromyographic component of the flexor reflex in 20 patients with complete and incomplete transversal spinal cord injuries. A marked, progressive, and prolonged decrease of both reflex components was observed in most patients. The early component was decreased less than the late reflex component immediately following the end of TENS, while further decrement of both components was observed 30 min after the end of TENS. The placebo stimulation in 4 patients revealed no decrease, or only a less marked decrease in reflex responses. So, he discussed that the marked suppressive effect of TENS could not be attributed to the potentiated habituation of the reflex responses alone and the induced inhibitory processes seemed to be at least partially localized at the segmental level of the spinal interneuron system.

Aydin et al. (2005) compared the efficacy of TENS with oral baclofen in the treatment of spastic SCI. Ten patients were assigned to oral baclofen and eleven patients to TENS. Twenty healthy individuals were allocated to a control group. TENS was applied once per day for 15 minutes to the tibial nerve for 15 days at a frequency of 100Hz and pulse duration of 100 msecs. The outcome measures are Spasm frequency scale, painful spasm scale, lower limb Ashworth score, clonus score, deep tendon reflex, plantar stimulation response score, H-reflex and functional disability score, and Functional Independent Measure (FIM). They found a significant improvement in lower limb Ashworth score, spasm frequency scale, deep tendon reflex score, functional disability score and FIM in the baclofen and TENS groups ($P = 0.020$, $P = 0.014$, $P = 0.025$, $P = 0.003$, and $P = 0.003$, respectively) after treatment. There was a significant decrease in H-reflex maximum amplitude in the TENS group ($P = 0.026$). The percentage change of baclofen in these outcome variables was no different from that of repeated application of TENS in immediate and long-term evaluation ($P > 0.05$). They concluded that TENS should be recommended as an adjacent treatment to stretch and range of motion exercises.

Chung and Cheng (2010) randomly assigned eighteen SCI subjects with spasticity over lower limbs to receive either 60 minutes of active TENS (0.25 ms, 100 Hz, 15 mA) for 60 minutes of placebo TENS over the common peroneal nerve. Composite Spasticity Score was used to assess the spasticity level of ankle plantar flexors immediately before and after TENS application. Composite Spasticity Score consisted of Achilles tendon jerks, resistance to full-range passive ankle dorsiflexion and ankle clonus. Significant reductions were shown in Composite Spasticity Score by 29.5% ($p = 0.017$), resistance to full-range passive ankle dorsiflexion by 31.0% ($p= 0.024$) and ankle clonus by 29.6% ($p = 0.023$) in the TENS group but these reductions were not found in the placebo TENS group. The between-group differences of both Composite Spasticity Score and resistance to full-range passive ankle dorsiflexion were significant ($p = 0.027$ and $p = 0.024$, respectively). They concluded that a single session of TENS could immediately reduce spasticity.

Oo WM (2014) studied the immediate and short-term efficacy of adding transcutaneous electrical nerve stimulation (TENS) to standardized physical therapy on subacute spasticity within 6 months of spinal cord injury after subjects (N=16) with clinically determined spasticity were randomly assigned to either the experimental group (n=8) or the control group (n=8). Sixty-minute sessions of TENS over the bilateral common peroneal nerves before 30 minutes of physical therapy for the experimental group and 30 minutes of physical therapy alone for the control group for the duration of 3 weeks The composite spasticity score, which included 3 subscores (ankle jerk, muscle tone, and ankle clonus scores), was used as the primary end point to assess plantar flexor spasticity. These subscores were designated as secondary end points. Serial evaluations were made at baseline before study entry and immediately after the first and last sessions in both groups.. All patients in both groups had access to standardized rehabilitation care.

On analysis for immediate effects, there was a significant reduction only in the composite spasticity score (mean difference, 1.75; 99% confidence interval [CI], 0.47-3.03; P=.002) in the experimental group, but no significant reduction was observed in all outcome variables in the control group. A significant difference in the composite spasticity score (1.63; 99% CI, 0.14-3.11; P=.006) was observed between the 2 groups. After 15 sessions of treatment, a significant reduction was determined in the composite spasticity score (2.75; 99% CI, 1.31-4.19; P<.001), the muscle tone score (1.75; 99% CI, 0.16-3.34; P=.006), and the ankle clonus score (0.75; 99% CI, 0.18-1.32; P=.003) in the experimental group, whereas none of the outcome variables revealed a significant reduction in the control group. The between-group difference was significant only for the composite spasticity score (2.13; 99% CI, 0.59-3.66; P=.001) and the muscle tone score (1.50; 99% CI, 0.15-2.85; P=.005) after 15 intervention sessions. The author concluded that addition of TENS to standardized physical therapy had synergistically antispastic action, providing more effective reduction of clinical spasticity.

In the review of electrical stimulation in the management of spasticity, Campbell (1998) remarked that electrical stimulation was safe in comparison with muscle weakness, depression of CNS associated with oral drugs, and risks of infection associated with implanted medication devices. Electrical stimulation should be the initial preferred management, compared with muscle weakness or complete denervation related with botulinum toxin and phenol nerve block.

Pharmacological Management

A variety of medications are available for the treatment of spasticity. When spasticity is focal rather than diffuse in nature, the sedation, confusion and muscle weakness associated with the use of oral medications may limit their effectiveness.

I) Oral Pharmacological Therapy

The specific pharmacologic effects can be directed toward alteration of transmitters by suppression of excitation (glutamate), enhancement of inhibition (GABA or glycine), a combination of noradrenaline (norepinephrine), serotonin, adenosine, and various neuropeptides, or action on peripheral neuromuscular sites. Although numerous substances have potential antispasticity effects, the USA Food and Drug Administration (FDA) has approved only four prescription pharmaceuticals for the treatment of spasticity related to central nervous system disorder. These are baclofen, tizanidine, dantrolene sodium, and diazepam (Nance et al., 2011).

Because oral medications produce systemic side-effects, they are usually used in patients with diffuse spasticity. As these medications produce non-targeted release of pharmacological agents, their major side-effect is a general suppression of neuronal activity in individuals who already have a reduced voluntary drive (Elbasiouny et al., 2010).

There is a level 1 evidence for oral baclofen, tazanidine and clonidine in spastic SCI patients. There is a lack of available evidence to support diazepam use as an adjunctive treatment to baclofen in persons with SCI. In head-to-head comparison studies, clonidine was superior to diazepam, and placebo but inferior to baclofen in reducing spasticity as measured by the H-reflex and vibration inhibition index (Hsieh et al., 2007).

Although level 1 evidence is also found for the ongoing use of cyproheptadine, gabapentin, and L-threo- nine for spasticity treatment secondary to SCI, reported therapeutic benefit was limited (Hsieh et al., 2007).

No current evidence (from 1980) could be found to support the use of dantrolene and diazepam in the treatment of spasticity secondary to SCI (Hsieh et al., 2007).

II) Chemical Neurolysis

Chemical neurolysis is usually used in individuals with focal spasticity. A peripheral nerve innervating spastic muscles is injected with phenol or alcohol solutions which destroy myelin. Aqueous phenol is also used for motor point injection in spastic muscles. However, the effectiveness of the injection diminishes over time and repeated injections are needed.

The potential complications of phenol or alcohol injection include pain, dysesthesias that can last from weeks to months, arrhythmias, variable duration of effect, and incomplete irreversibility. Subarachnoid block has been performed with intrathecal phenol or alcohol, although this therapy can result in severe weakness and reduced sphincter (Nance et al., 2011).

III) Botulinum Injection

Botulinum toxin, injected intramuscularly, acts on the neuromuscular junction to inhibit the release of acetylcholine. The toxin causes chemical denervation of intrafusal and extrafusal muscle fibers, and its effect is reversible. The treatment is effective in reducing pain and muscle spasm. The major side effect is excessive weakness of the treated muscle (Nance et al., 2011).

There is level 4 evidence that botulinum neurotoxin improves focal muscle spasticity secondary to SCI (Hsieh et al., 2007).

IV) Intrathecal Baclofen Infusion

The intrathecal route of baclofen administration results in a marked increase (100 times) in potency compared to the oral treatment. The implantable drug delivery system is used for chronic slow infusion into the intrathecal space. Several studies have demonstrated the effectiveness of intrathecal baclofen for the treatment of spasticity.

This treatment is limited by the invasive nature of the treatment and the cost of the implantable devices (Nance et al., 2011).

Only level 4 evidence supports the use of intrathecal baclofen for long-term maintainance of spasticity, improved functional outcomes, low complications rates, and cost-effectiveness (Hsieh et al., 2007).

Surgical Interventions

Orthopedics and neurosurgery are commonly involved in the treatment of spasticity. Common goals of surgery are usually to increase mobility, to decrease the use of external aids, to correct or prevent deformity, and ultimately to maximize function.

Orthopedic surgeons use musculoskeletal compensatory techniques such as tendon lengthening, muscle-tendon transfer, contracture release, capsulotomy, osteotomy, resection arthroplasty, arthrodesis, epiphyseodesis, ankle fusion, and spine fusion.

The neurosurgeons use the neuroablative techniques such as interruption of the spinal reflex arc by neurectomy, neurotomy, rhizotomy, selective rhizotomy, dorsal root entry zone lesion, and myelotomy. Other procedures include cordotomy, cordectomy, implantation of stimulators, or drug infusion devices (Nance et al., 2011).

Intractable spasticity refractive to conservative approaches can be treated by dorsal Tmyelotomy (Poupre's technique is more effective than the Bischof II) as supported by level 2 evidence (Hsieh et al., 2007).

REFERENCES

Adams MM and Hicks AL (2005). Spasticity after spinal cord injury. *Spinal Cord* 2005; 43, 577–586.

Ashworth B (1964). Preliminary trial of carisoprodol in multiple sclerosis. *Practitioner* 1964; 192: 540–542.

Aydin G, Tomruk S, Keles I, Demir SO and Orkun S (2005). Transcutaneous electrical nerve stimulation versus baclofen in spasticity: clinical and electrophysiologic comparison. *Am J Phys Med Rehabil* 2005; 84: 584-592.

Bajd T and Vodovnik L (1984). Pendulum testing of spasticity. *J Biomed Eng*, 6: 9–16.

Bandi S and Ward AB (2010). Spasticity. International Encyclopedia of Rehabilitation

Barnes MP (1998). Review: Management of spasticity. Age *and Ageing 1998;* 27: 239-245.

Bavikatte G and Gaber T (2009). Approach to spasticity in general practice. *BJMP*. 2009:2(3) 29-34

Beres-Jones JA, Johnson TD, Harkem SJ (2003). Clonus after human spinal cord injury cannot be attributed solely to recurrent muscle-tendon stretch. *Exp Brain Res*. 2003 Mar ;149 (2):222-36.

Biering-Sørensen F, Nielsen JB and Klinge K (2006). Spasticity-assessment: a review. *Spinal Cord*. 2006 Dec;44(12):708-22.

Bohannon RW and Smith MB (1987). Interrater reliability of a modified Ashworth scale of muscle spasticity. *Phys Ther* 1987; 67: 206–207.

Boorman GI, Lee RG, Becker WJ and Windhorst UR (1996). Impaired "natural reciprocal inhibition" in patients with spasticity due to incomplete spinal cord injury. *Electroencephalogr Clin Neurophysiol* 1996; 101(2): 84-92.

Bucy PC, Kephnger JE and Siqucira EB (1964). Destruction of the pyramidal tract in man. *J. Neurosurg.* 21, 385–398.

Burke D and Ashby P (1972). Are spinal 'presynaptic' inhibitory mechanisms suppressed in spascity? *J. Neurol. Sci.* 15, 321–326.

Campbell JM (1998). Electrical stimulation in the management of spasticity. http://media.kenanaonline.com/files/0017/17204/campbell.pdf accessed 21 May 2011.

Carpenter RHS (1984). *Neurophysiology.* London: Arnold Heinmann, p. 234.

Chung BPH and Cheng BKK (2010). Immediate effect of transcutaneous electrical nerve stimulation on spasticity in patients with spinal cord injury. *Clin Rehabil* 2010; 24: 202-210.

Cooper G (2006). *Essential Physical Medicine and Rehabilitation.* Humana Press, Totowa, New Jersy, pp. 59-100.

Crone C, Johnsen LL, Biering-Sorensen F and Nielsen JB (2003). Appearance of reciprocal facilitation of ankle extensors from ankle flexors in patients with stroke or spinal cord injury. *Brain* 2003; 126: 495-507.

Davidoff RA (1992). Skeletal muscle tone and the misunderstood stretch reflex. *Neurology* 1992; 42(5):951-63.

Decq P (2003) Pathophysiology of spasticity. *Neurochirurgie* 2003; 49: 163-184.

Delwaide PJ (1993). Pathophysiological mechanisms of spasticity at the spinal cord level. In: Thilmann AF, Burke DJ and Rymer WZ (eds), *Spasticity: Mechanisms and Management.* Heidelberg, Germany: Springer-Verlag; 1993:296-308.

Delwaide PJ and Pennisi G (1994). Tizanidine and electrophysiologic analysis of spinal control mechanisms in humans with spasticity. *Neurology*, 44 (suppl. 9): S21–8.

Dietz V, Quintern J and Berger W (1981). Electrophysiological studies of gait in spasticity and rigidity. Evidence that altered mechanical properties of muscle contribute to hypertonia. *Brain* 104, 431–449.

Dimitrijevic MR, Nathan PW, Sherwood AMJ (1980). Clonus: the role of central mechanisms. *Neurol Neurosurg Psychiatry.* 1980 Apr;43(4):321-32.

Ditunno JF, Little JW, Tessler A and Burns AS (2004). Spinal shock revisited: a four-phase model. *Spinal Cord* (2004) 42, 383-395.

Elbasiouny S, Moroz D, Bakr M and. Mushahwar V (2010). Management of spasticity after spinal cord injury: current techniques and future directions. *Neurorehabil Neural Repair* 2010; 24: 23-33.

Elovic E and Baerga E (2004). Spasticity. In: SJ Cuccurullo (ed), *Physical Medicine and Rehabilitation Board Review*, 3 rd edn, Demos Medical Publishing, New York, pp. 743-749.

Elovic EP, Eisenberg ME and Jasay NN,Jr (2010). Spasticity and muscle overactivity as components of upper motor neurone syndrome. In: JA Delisa and BM Gans (eds), *Physical Medicine & Rehabilitation: Principles and Practice.* 5th edn, Lippincott Williams & Wilkins, pp. 1319-1344.

Faist M, Mazevet D, Dietz V and Pierrot-Deseilligny E (1994). A quantitative assessment of presynaptic inhibition of la afferents in spastics: differences in hemiplegics and paraplegics. *Brain* 1994; 117(6): 1449-1455.

Fisher CM, and Curry HB (1965). Pure motor hemiplegia of vascular origin. *Arch. Neurol.* 13, 30–44.

Fleuren JFM (2009). *Assessment of spasticity, from EMG to patient's perception.* doctoral thesis, the University of Twente, Enschede, The Netherlands.

Fries W, Danek A, Schidumann K, and Hamburger C (1993). Motor recovery following capsular stroke. Role of descending pathways from multiple motor areas. *Brain* 116, 369–382.

Ganong WF (2010). *Review Of Medical Physiology*, 23rd edn, Appleton and Lange, Stamford, pp. 115-129.

Gorassini MA, Knash ME, Harvey PJ, Bennett DJ and Yang JF (2004). Role of motoneurons in the generation of muscle spasms after spinal cord injury. *Brain* 2004; 127: 2247-2258.

Goulet C, Arsenault AB, Bourbonnais D, Laramée MT and Lepage Y (1996). Effects of transcutaneous electrical nerve stimulation on H-reflex and spinal spasticity. *Scand J Rehabil Med* 1996; 28(3): 169-176.

Gracies JM (2005a). Pathophysiology of spastic paresis. I: Paresis and soft tissue changes. *Muscle Nerve* 31, 535–551.

Gracies JM (2005b). Pathophysiology of spastic paresis. II: Emergence of muscle overactivity. *Muscle Nerve* 31, 552–571.

Gregoric M (1998). Suppression of flexor reflex by transcutaneous electrical nerve stimulation in spinal cord injured patients. *Muscle Nerve* 1998; 21: 166-172.

Hagbarth KE, Wallin G and Lofstedt L (1973). Muscle spindle responses to stretch in normal and spastic subjects. *Scand J Rehabil Med.* 1973;5: 156-159.

Hagbarth, K. E., Hagglund, J. V., Nordin, M. & Wallin, E. U. (1985). Thixotropic behaviour of human finger flexor muscles with accompanying changes in spindle and reflex responses to stretch. *J Physiol (Lond)*, 368: 323–42.

Hammar I and Jankowska E (2003). Modulatory effects of alpha 1-, alpha 2-, and beta-receptor agonists on feline spinal interneurons with monosynaptic input from group I muscle afferents. *J Neurosci* 2003; 23: 332-338.

Han JS, Chen XH, Yuan Y and Yan SC (1994). Transcutaneous electrical nerve stimulation for treatment of spinal spasticity. *Chin Med J (Engl)* 1994; 107(1): 6-11.

Hiersemenzel LP, Curt A and Dietz V (2000). From spinal shock to spasticity: neuronal adaptations to a spinal cord injury. *Neurology* 2000; 54(8): 1574-1582.

Hsieh JTC, Wolfe DL, Connolly S, Townson AF, Curt A, Blackmer J, Sequeira K, Aubut J (2007). Spasticity after spinal cord injury: anEvidence-Based Review of Current Interventions. *Top Spinal Cord Inj Rehabil* 2007;13(1):81–97

Hsieh JT, Wolfe DL, Miller WC and Curt A (2008). Spasticity outcome measures in spinal cord injury: psychometric properties and clinical utility. *Spinal Cord.* 2008 Feb;46(2):86-95.

Hultborn H, Illert M and Santini M (1976). Convergence on interneurones mediating the reciprocal la inhibition of motoneurons. III. Effects from supraspinal pathways. *Acta Physiol. Scand.* 96, 368–391.

Jankowska E and Roberts W J (1972). Synaptic actions of single interneurons mediating reciprocal la inhibition of motoneurons. *J. Physiol. (Lond)* 222, 623– 642.

Johnson GR and Pandyan AD (2008). The Measurement of spasticity. In: MP Barnes and GR Johnson (ed), *Upper Motor Neurone and Spasticity*, Cambridge University Press, New York, pp. 64-78.

Kirshblum S and Brooks M (2010). Rehabilitation of spinal cord injury. In: JA Delisa and BM Gans (eds), *Physical Medicine & Rehabilitation: Principles and Practice*. 5th edn, Lippincott Williams & Wilkins, pp. 665-716.

Lance JW (1980). Symposium synopsis. In: RG Feldman, RR Young & WW Koella (eds), *Spasticity: Disordered Motor Control. Symposia Specialists, Miami* (1980), pp. 485–500. Year Book Medical Publishers, Chicago.

Levin MF, Hui-Chan CW (1992). Relief of hemiparetic spasticity by TENS is associated with improvement in reflex and voluntary motor functions. *Electroencephalogr Clin Neurophysiol* 1992; 85(2): 131-142.

Li S, Kamper DG and Rymer WZ (2006). Effects of changing wrist positions on finger flexor hypertonia in stroke survivors. *Muscle Nerve*, 33: 183–90.

Lundberg A (1975). Control of spinal mechanism from the brain. In: D. Tower and R. Brady (eds), *The Nervous System,* Vol. 1, New York: Raven Press, 253–265.

Lundberg A (1979). Multisensory control of spinal reflex pathways. *Prog. Brain Res.* 50, 11–28.

Malhotra S, Pandyan AD, Day CR, Jones PW and Hermens H (2009). Spasticity, an impairment that is poorly defined and poorly measured. *Clin Rehabil* 2009; 23: 651-658.

Malouin, F., Bonneau, C., Pichard, L. & Corriveau, D. (1997). Non-reflex mediated changes in plantarflexor muscles early after stroke. *Scand J Rehabil* Med, 29: 147–53.

Milanov I and Georgiev D (1994). Mechanisms of tizanidineaction on spasticity. *Acta Neurol Scand*, 89: 274–9.

Miller L, Mattison P, Paul L and Wood L (2007). The effects of transcutaneous electrical nerve stimulation (TENS) on spasticity in multiple sclerosis. *Mult scler* 2007; 13: 527-533.

McCouch GP, Austin GM, Liu CN and Liu CY (1958). Sprouting as a cause of spasticity. *J Neurophysiol.* 1958;21:205-216.

Mukherjee A and Chakravarty A. 2010. Spasticity mechanisms – for the clinician. Frontiers in neurology 01/2010; 1:149.

Nadeau S, Goulet C, Arsenault AB, Gravel D, Bourbonnais D, Lepage Y (1999). Assessment of the plantarflexor muscle tone in chronic stroke and spinal cord injury subjects using the spasticity index. *Neurorehabil Neural Repair* 1999; 13: 57.

Nance PW (2003). Management of spasticity. In: VW Lin (ed), *Spinal Cord Medicine Principle and Prictice*, Demos Medical Publishing, New York, pp. 461-476.

Nance PW and Satkunam L and Ethans K (2011). Spasticity management. In: RL Braddom (ed), *Physical Medicine and Rehabilitation*, 4th edn, W.B. Saunders Company, Philadelphiea, pp. 638-656.

Nielsen JF and Sinkjaer T (1996). A comparison of clinical and laboratory measures of spasticity. *Mult Scler* 1996; 1(5): 296-301.

Neptune RR,Burnfield JM and Mulroy SJ (2007). The neuromuscular demands of toe walking: A forward dynamics simuation analysis. Journal of Biomechanics 2007; 40: 1293-1300.

Nielsen JB, Crone C and Hultborn H (2007). The spinal pathophysiology of spasticity – from a basic science point of view. *Acta Physiol* 2007, 189, 171–180.

Oo WM (2014). Efficacy of addition of transcutaneous electrical nerve stimulation to standardized physical therapy in subacute spinal spasticity: a randomized controlled trial. Arch Phys Med Rehabil 2014 Nov;95(11):2013-20.

Patel DR. (2005). Therapeutic interventions in cerebral palsy. *Indian J Pediatr*. 72(11), 979-983.

Penn RD, Savoy SM, Corcos D, Latash M, Gottlieb G and Parke B. (1989). Intrathecal baclofen for severe spinal spasticity. *N Engl J Med* 1989; 320: 1517–1521.

Pompetano O (1984). Recurrent inhibition. In: F. A. Davidoff (ed), *Handbook of the Spinal Cord,* Vols. 2 and 3, New York: Marcel Dekker Press, 461–557.

Priebe MM, Sherwood AM, Thornby JI, Kharas NF and Markowski J (1996). Clinical assessment of spasticity in spinal cord injury: a multidimensional problem. *Arch Phys Med Rehabil* 1996; 77: 713–716.

Rossi A, Maocchio R and Scarpini C (1990). Clonus in man: a rhythmic oscillation maintained by a reflex mechanism. *Electroencephalogr Clin Neurophysiol* 75:56–63.

Rothwell JC (1994). Investigating reflex pathways and their function. In: *Control of Human Voluntary Movement*, 2nd edn. London: Chapman & Hall, pp. 153– 212.

Sawynok J and Reid A (1994). Spinal supersensitivity to 5-HT1, 5- HT2 and 5- HT3 receptor agonists following 5,7-dihydroxytryptamine. *Eur J Pharmacol* 1994; 264: 249–257.

Schindler-Ivens SM and Shields RK (2004). Soleus H-reflex recruitment is not altered in persons with chronic spinal cord injury. *Arch Phys Med Rehabil* 85, 840–847.

Schmidt RF (1971). Presynaptic inhibition in the vertebrate central nervous system. *Ergeb. Physiol.* 63, 91–101.

Schomburg ED, Steffens H (1998). The effect of DOPA and clonidine on reflex pathways from group II afferents to alpha-motoneurones in the cat. *Exp Brain Res* 71; 442-446,

Shahani BT, and Young RR (1973). Human flexor spasm. In: J. E. Desmedt (ed) *New Developments in Electromyography and Clinical Neurophysiology*, Vol. 3, Basal: S Karger AG, 734–743.

Sheean G (2008). Neurophysiology of spasticity. In: MP Barnes and GR Johnson (ed), *Upper Motor Neurone and Spasticity*, Cambridge University Press, New York, pp. 9-63.

Shefner JM, Berman SA, Sarkarati M and Young RR (1992). Recurrent inhibition is increased in patients with spinal cord injury. *Neurology* 42, 2162–2168.

Sherwood AM, Graves DE and Priebe MM (2000). Altered motor control and spasticity after spinal cord injury: subjective and objective assessment. *J Rehabil Res Dev* 2000; 37: 41–52.

Sköld C, Levi R and Seiger A (1999). Spasticity after traumatic spinal cord injury: nature, severity, and location. *Arch Phys Med Rehabil* 1999; 80: 1548–1557.

Steeves JD, Lammertse D, Curt A, Fawcett JW, Tuszynski MH and Ditunno JF (2007). Guidelines for the conduct of clinical trials for spinal cord injury (SCI) as developed by the ICCP panel: clinical trial outcome measures. *Spinal Cord* 2007; 45: 206–221.

Thilmann AF, Fellows SJ and Garms E (1991a). The mechanism of spastic muscle hypertonus. *Brain*, 114: 233–44.

Vanek ZF (2010). Spasticity introduction and pathophysiology. http:// emedicine. medscape.com/article/1148826-overview#showall accessed 19 Jan 2015.

Voerman GE, Gregoric M. and Hermens H (2005). Neurophysiological methods for the assessment of spasticity: the Hoffmann reflex, the tendon reflex, and the stretch reflex. *Disabil Rehabil*, 27: 33–68.

Walsh, E. G. (1992). Muscles, masses and motion: the physiology of normality, hypotonicity, spasticity and rigidity. In: *Clinics in Developmental Medicine, no. 125*. Oxford: Blackwell Scientific/Mac Keith Press, pp. 78– 102.

Ward AB and Javaid S (2008). Pharmacological management of spasticity. In: MP Barnes and GR Johnson (ed), *Upper Motor Neurone and Spasticity*, Cambridge University Press, New York, pp. 131-149.

Wartenberg R (1951). Pendulousness of the legs as a diagnostic test. *Neurology* 1951; 1: 1824.

Walsh DM and Basford JR (2009). Transcutaneous Electrical Nerve Stimulation. In: HS Smith (ed), *Current Therapy in Pain*, Elsevier, pp. 541-546.

Yang J, Fung J, Edamura M, Blunt R, Stein R and Barbeau H (1991). H-reflex modulation during walking in spastic paretic subjects. *Can J Neurol Sci.* 1991;18:443-452.

INDEX

C

D

G

H

I

J

K

L

M

N

O

P

Q

R

S

T

U

V

W

Z